Anti-Ageing Medicines

Marios Kyriazis M.D.

16pt

9781459665927

Read How You Want
LARGE PRINT BOOKS, BRAILLE & DAISY

Copyright Page from the Original Book

This edition published in the UK in 2005
by Watkins Publishing, Sixth Floor, Castle House,
75-76 Wells Street, London W1T 3QH

Some of the material included in this book originally appeared in *Carnosine and Other Elixirs of Youth*
ISBN 1 84293 049 4

This book is not to be used as a substitute for professional medical care and treatment. The ultimate decision concerning care should be between you and your doctor. The information in this book is offered with no guarantees on the part of the author and Publisher.

Designed and typeset by Jerry Goldie Graphic Design Printed and bound in Great Britain

Library of Congress Cataloging in Publication data available

ISBN 978 1 780283 00 5

www.watkinspublishing.com

TABLE OF CONTENTS

Dr Marios Kyriazis is an internationally acclaimed pioneer in the science and application of anti-ageing medicine. He is a practising physician who has also studied gerontology (the science of ageing) at King's College, University of London. He has a Diploma in Geriatric Medicine from the Royal College of Physicians of London and he is a Chartered Biologist and member of the Institute of Biology for work into the biology of ageing.

He is the founder of The British Longevity Society and is an advisor to several other age-related organisations. He has published over 400 articles on healthy ageing, both for scientists and for the public.

BY THE SAME AUTHOR

The Anti-Ageing Plan
Stay Young Longer – Naturally
The Look Young Bible
Carnosine and Other Elixirs of Youth

To Stella

ACKNOWLEDGEMENTS

I would like to express my thanks to the following who helped in one way or another:

Professor Alexander Boldyrev of the Lomonosov Moscow State University, for support and advice; Dr Mark Babizhayev for providing details about the ophthalmic uses of carnosine; Dr Alan Hipkiss, of the University of London, for useful discussions; Dr Jay Olshansky, of the University of Illinois, for criticising some of the issues surrounding anti-ageing treatments; International Anti-Aging Systems for providing the carnosine and for initiating dialogue; also for their permission to use material on calorie restriction mimetics, originally published in the *Anti-Aging Bulletin* with myself as an author.

Introduction

This book offers you the chance to learn something about the intricacies of the ageing process, and to get some 'inside' information on how ageing can affect you. I will start by explaining some of the simple concepts, and then tackle in earnest some of the dark and difficult to understand aspects of ageing. My aims are simple and practical. The first is to discuss and explain the actions of the most important anti-ageing remedies available today, highlighting both their benefits and their shortcomings. My second aim is, by explaining the many puzzling details of the ageing process, to provide you with enough knowledge to enable you, with the help of your physician, to choose your medication purposefully and effectively.

Before I discuss the benefits of these agents, we need to explore in some detail the basics of the ageing process. I do not assume that you have any previous knowledge of the subject, but I will gradually go into it in sufficient depth to stimulate the interest even of those with a relatively advanced understanding of ageing. Let me start by answering a few questions people may have about ageing.

WHAT IS AGEING?

The prestigious scientific journal, *Biogerontology,* defines ageing as: 'The progressive failing ability of the body's own intrinsic and genetic powers to defend, maintain and repair itself in order to keep on working efficiently'.

Traditional scientists believe ageing to be a natural phenomenon which is:

- intrinsic (in our genes)
- deleterious (detrimental with no benefits)
- universal (affecting every living thing)
- progressive (going only in one direction and irreversible).

Cutting-edge thinking, however, shows that this view is becoming difficult to support. Although ageing is indeed written into our genes, it is not completely irreversible. The clock has been turned back in a number of pioneering experiments during the past few years and, on at least one occasion involving groundbreaking cloning techniques, it has been reset to zero.

Ageing is certainly not due to a simple lack of a hormone or nutrient. Taking supplements or replacing a single nutrient is not going to reverse ageing. It is a much more complicated process than that, and there are several different mechanisms involved in it. Some of these mechanisms overlap, others are independent, but all of them are complicated. Any book trying to explain ageing for lay people is bound to be simplistic so, if you do find the following discussion difficult, bear in mind that in real life things are even more complex than this.

IS AGEING A DISEASE?

The simple answer is 'no'. Contrary to what many people – including some doctors and scientists – believe, ageing is not a disease.

Consider the following common condition – someone who, because of their age, is unable to talk properly, too weak to walk and confined to bed, with a severely reduced sense of balance, unable to feed themselves and relying on the care of others, they are incontinent of urine and faeces, and have a very poor memory. Is this person ill? Of course not, I am talking about a baby here. This baby may or may not have an illness which affects babies, such as nappy (diaper) rash or abdominal colic, but it is not ill merely because it has the characteristics of a baby.

It is the same with ageing. Ageing as such is not a disease, but just another period in our normal life. There are diseases which can affect anybody but which are, in fact, more common in later life – such as strokes and heart disease, diabetes, certain types of cancers, dementia, osteoporosis and arthritis. Young children can also have arthritis or cancer, teenagers can have diabetes, and twenty-year-olds can die of a heart attack. These are illnesses, and should not be confused with the natural underlying process of ageing. Ageing is a natural phenomenon and it is a progressive inability of the body to maintain and repair itself. Fighting age-related illness is one thing, fighting the ageing process is another. Having said that, however, many natural ageing mechanisms frequently result in actual diseases, so fighting an ageing process may well bring about an improvement of an age-related illness.

Ageing has been a fact of life since life was first created. All animals or plants, even if they are protected from an early death caused by predators or disease, will eventually show signs of ageing. Many people use chemicals extracted from plants to help them ward off the signs of ageing. Have you ever wondered why we have this natural inclination to choose plant chemicals in our fight against illness? Nature created these plant chemicals with the sole aim of protecting plants against disease or ageing. Humans came along afterwards and adapted these chemicals for their own use, to increase their chances of maintaining their health.

Humans have always been able to live for many years and also to experience at least some of the signs of ageing. During certain periods of human evolution, ageing was only experienced by very few people, and then only a small minority of those people lived to a very old age. Nowadays, many more people live to reach 'old age' (75–80 years) and even more live to a 'very old age' (90–100 years). The average lifespan is, as we know, increasing.

Surprisingly, there are still respectable scientists out there who believe that the average human lifespan cannot increase any more. They believe that it would be impossible for most people to live to the age of 85 or more. I remember how in the 1970s scientists were claiming that the average lifespan simply could not be extended beyond 80 years of age. Now that this limit is being reached, these scientists have changed their position and increased their estimate to 85 years of age. In a few years they will probably change their minds again and increase the limit to 90. In fact, there are other equally respectable scientists who claim that, with time and effort, it will be possible to extend the average human lifespan to around 110–120 years: that is to reach the maximum limit of a natural lifespan.

Beyond that age, the estimates and speculation enter the realms of science fiction, and so I am not going to discuss this further. People who claim that we will be able to live to an age of 200 and beyond, are simply looking too far into the future in a way that is not relevant to us, our children or our grandchildren. Perhaps genetic science, biotechnology and bioengineering will make the steps that are necessary for people to achieve that unnatural age, but this is not going to happen in our time or during the next generation. I just want to highlight the fact that a respectable Cambridge scientist, Aubrey De Grey, believes that by the year 2100 our life expectancy will be 5000 years!

WHAT IS ANTI-AGEING MEDICINE?

Anti-ageing medicine is a branch of medical science and applied medicine, aimed at treating the underlying causes of ageing and at alleviating any age-related ailment, with the ultimate goal of extending the healthy lifespan of humans. It aims not only to prevent and reduce the severity of age-related diseases – arthritis, dementia, cataracts for example – but also to prevent and reduce the severity of ailments which are due to the natural process of ageing, such as skin ageing, and the loss of muscle tissue, and so maintain some of the characteristics of youth.

It uses conventional and alternative regimes in an integrated approach to achieve the best possible result for the patient. It is a holistic discipline, seeing the patient as a whole and not just as an isolated disease. Perhaps one of the most important characteristics of anti-ageing medicine is that it is not so much concerned with treating existing diseases, but rather with preventing future age-related health problems.

Many people claim to be experts in anti-ageing medicine, when in fact they have not had any suitable training. Some are not even medical practitioners. Others use the term 'anti-ageing medicine' rather liberally to include quack treatments and therapies which have no scientific basis whatsoever. Interested individuals can study age-related medicine at accredited universities, and there are also other courses of study, for example those offered by the American Academy of Anti-Aging Medicine, which is, however, not formally accredited by the medical profession.

Anti-ageing medicine is not merely geriatric medicine. Geriatric medicine is the treatment of old people who are ill, whereas anti-ageing medicine is aimed at both young and old people who want to prevent age-related problems for as long as possible, and to maintain health into old age. According to one of the first modern anti-ageing physicians, the Romanian Professor Ana Aslan, treating ageing is both 'a science and an art'.

Some scientists and doctors are uncomfortable with the term 'anti-ageing medicine', because they think it is unscientific. They suggest more scientific-sounding terms such as 'interventive biogerontology' or even 'strategies for engineered negligible senescence (SENSe)'. The latter term basically means to artificially slow down ageing to almost zero. These terms may have relevance in scientific circles but they do not change the general meaning of what anti-ageing medicine is. My grandmother used to say, 'John is still John, no matter how he dresses.' You can change the terminology as much as you like, but the underlying essence of anti-ageing medicine will remain the same.

WHAT IS YOUTH?

Youth, in the context of anti-ageing medicine, is taken to mean not merely not being old, but possessing some, or all, of the characteristics of idealized youth, for example:

- good health
- strong muscles
- an efficient immune system
- a sharp memory and a healthy brain
- hormones working at their peak capacity

It does not matter how old you actually are: in other words, it is not a matter of chronological age, but a matter of improving a person's biological, social, spiritual and mental state. Somebody is considered 'aged' or 'old' who has succumbed to the problems related to age. You may be of an advanced chronological age but still retain some of the characteristics of youth. For example, there are 90-year-olds who look healthy, are without any significant illnesses, feel energetic and enjoy life to the full. They are content and fulfilled, and enjoy the best of both worlds – the health of youth plus the wisdom of age.

Anti-ageing medicine is not necessarily directed against all ageing as such, but only against the medical or health problems of ageing. Some aspects of ageing can be really beneficial. For example, wisdom and understanding of the world increase with age, spiritual matters are better appreciated, and there are even some physical areas which improve with age:

- allergies generally become less troublesome
- travel sickness is less likely to occur
- sensitivity to pain decreases.

By the same token, youth is not necessarily a totally good thing, and certain aspects of it – such as health and a youthful appearance – are more desirable than others. Inexperience and insecurity, for example, are definitely seen as undesirable in the eyes of many older people. Youth should not be confused with a young chronological age. What most people are trying to achieve is not a young chronological age but a young biological age – they want to be healthy and biologically efficient.

WHAT IS AN ELIXIR OF YOUTH?

An elixir, disregarding the mythical, alchemical and unscientific connotations, is a solution or mixture of chemicals used as a medicine or for treatment. There is a subtle difference between 'the elixir of life' (a preparation which is intended to prolong life indefinitely) and the 'elixir of youth' (a preparation which can maintain youth as defined above). In this book I am not talking about prolonging life indefinitely but about prolonging some of the characteristics of youth.

WORDS

A lot of people, including some respectable scientists, are in a muddle about the different terms used in the anti-ageing field. They use words like 'longevity', 'immortality' and 'rejuvenation' without making a distinction between them. These words may sound as if they refer to similar things but there is, in fact, a great difference between them. Any linguist will tell you that 'longevity' simply means 'long life'. An anti-ageing physician will tell you that longevity does not mean merely prolonging life for the sake of it, but also extending the number of years you can live in good health. Those who are opposed to pursuing longevity, thinking that its aim is merely to add years to life, irrespective of all the illnesses that come with that, are simply mistaken. 'Longevity', in the eyes of an anti-ageing practitioner, is not one, but two things – living longer and being healthier.

You will notice that when I speak of 'living longer' I am not specific and do not refer to any numbers. How much longer? Longer than what? The answers are vague. By as much as possible. Longer than others. I think by 'a long life' most people mean an age of 90–95 years, whereas a minority may mean an age of over 100.

Other terms used in the anti-ageing field are:

- ‘rejuvenation’ which means ‘to make young again’
- ‘eternal life’ means living forever. ‘Forever’ can, however,
- mean different things for different people. Some take it to mean 200–300 years of age, whereas others consider it to mean 1000 years. Some people take it literally, really forever.
- ‘immortality’ means never dying, which is, in a sense, similar to the above terms.

Notice that none of the above terms says anything about being healthy or unhealthy. They should be used correctly and not too literally. Treatment with a certain product will not make you ‘immortal’, but may grant you a certain degree of ‘longevity’. Future treatment with genetic manipulation may bring about ‘rejuvenation’ but not ‘eternal life’.

ANIMAL EXPERIMENTS

In this book I refer extensively to research done not only on cells in the laboratory but also to experiments performed on animals such as rats, mice, dogs, and rabbits. If you are seriously against animal experimentation then you will need to decide whether this book is for you or not. Whether I oppose or support animal experiments is not a relevant issue here. I am merely reporting on what other people have already done. My own experiments are based solely on consenting human volunteers, who are fully informed about their treatment.

There is an important distinction to be made between results based on animal studies and those based on studies with humans. The majority of the results presented in this book are based on animal studies. Although there are certain biological similarities between animals and humans, this does not mean that a positive result from an animal study will necessarily hold true for humans as well. Many, if not all, manufacturers of anti-ageing products quote positive research results but they do not always make a distinction between animal and human research.

In many situations, animal research can help us to better understand ourselves, and lays the foundations for human experiments. Quite often the human studies happen to agree with results from animal studies but this is by no means always the case. So I would warn you against being taken in by enthusiastic advertisements, which claim positive findings unless these have been shown to be true specifically for humans.

Any type of scientific research, even research published in established, prestigious journals, can easily be criticized and flaws can be found. At university we were given classic excerpts from scientific articles (such as those describing the discovery of DNA) and asked to find flaws in them, as an exercise. We were always successful. People who are opposed to anti-ageing medicine may criticize some of the studies mentioned in this book. This is nothing unusual, it is an established scientific practice. The studies are presented as a whole, to give a sense of the general direction of the research and are not to be taken in isolation or at face value.

There is a difference between an 'experiment' and a 'clinical trial'. An experiment is when a treatment or a procedure is tried on animals or humans in artificial and controlled surroundings. A clinical trial is when a drug treatment is given to human patients, in real situations, who are then monitored to see what happens to them. For the sake of simplicity, I use these two terms without making a distinction.

PIONEERING TREATMENTS

All of the treatments referred to in this book form part of anti-ageing medicine, which is a new and pioneering medical discipline. By definition, pioneering means that we are not sure what is over the horizon. It is inevitable that there will be a degree of speculation and conjecture as well as uncertainties, contradictions and uncorroborated evidence regarding the treatments. Anti-ageing medicine is still not a fully established discipline, and if you decide to use its treatments you should understand that nothing is guaranteed, at least not in the sense of traditional, established medical disciplines. You should be willing to be flexible, tolerant, open-minded and curious to find out more about a particular drug.

An important point is that, whereas research may not yet fully support the use of a product, this product may actually work for you as an individual. On the other hand, research may support the use of a product which happens not to be particularly effective for you. So it is a matter of personal experimentation, trial and error, based on what current science has to offer.

USING ANTI-AGEING DRUGS OR SUPPLEMENTS

I take it as a given that people who want to use any of the supplements or drugs referred to in this book, will only do so under medical or expert supervision. Some of the drugs mentioned are only available on a doctor's prescription, but others are not. There is no point in taking anti-ageing medicines without a clearly defined personalized plan which takes into account your own particular requirements, any illnesses or medical conditions, other drugs you may be taking, your lifestyle and any other relevant factors. The dose of each of these medicines needs to be adjusted depending on the individual, and only a specialist practitioner will have the necessary expertise to create a personalized plan for you. Taking anti-ageing medicines without expert supervision is not only a waste of money but you must be aware that it could also be dangerous.

AGEING AND WHAT CAUSES IT

There are several theories about what causes ageing. Some of these contradict each other, whereas some others overlap. Some make logical sense, whereas others do not. During a recent anti-ageing conference, we were ten people on a panel, drawn from a wide variety of scientific backgrounds, to answer questions from the audience. Towards the end of the session, one participant asked each one of us the simple question, 'What causes ageing?' The answer was not simple. In fact, there were ten almost completely different answers.

For the purpose of understanding ageing and making better sense of the treatments available I am going to concentrate on only a small number of the relevant theories. These not only make some sense but have an important plus – they give you the chance of doing something practical about your own ageing. These theories do not depend on some scientist using genetic engineering to extend the lifespan of fruit flies or worms, they do not depend on a high-tech company researching gene manipulation, and they are not about dull scientists churning out theoretical and academic jargon. The theories are based on practical, down-to-earth concepts which can easily be adapted and employed by anybody, in an attempt to enjoy a healthy life for as long as possible.

There are three main biochemical processes involved in ageing. These are oxidation, glycation and methylation. Other processes which can also have practical relevance are those involved in chronic inflammation or hormonal deregulation. The following is a very simple introduction to the biology of ageing, examining these processes.

OXIDATION

Most people have heard about the mayhem free radicals cause to your body. Free radicals are a group of simple compounds with an electron missing from their chemical structure and this makes them unstable. They seek out other chemical structures from which they can acquire an electron.

Free radicals are like single men at a married ladies' party. A single man at such a party would not just sit quietly looking out of the window, but would try to find a partner from the abundance of women available. When that single man did find a partner, it would mean that the husband of that woman would be without a wife, he would be angry and would go on to cause trouble, quite understandably. The party would end in disaster. This is exactly what happens when a free radical reacts with your tissues, causing a lot of heavy and permanent damage, leaving your body as devastated as a party which ended in a serious fight.

To be fair, free radicals in small and controlled quantities are useful in your everyday metabolism. They take part in several normal reactions within the body and they help you to breathe and consequently to live. The majority of free radicals are produced during oxygen metabolism, within your cells. When production of these free radicals increases and goes out of control, then the problems start.

One old proverb says that you are better able to fight your enemies if you give them a name. So here are the names of some free radicals:

- superoxide radicals
- hydrogen peroxide
- hydroxyl radicals
- nitric oxide

The scientific names for some of the different types of free radicals are reactive oxygen species (ROS, or oxygen free radicals), reactive nitrogen species (RNS, or nitrogen free radicals) and so on.

The human body has developed several effective ways of dealing with these troublemakers. Examples of these methods of defence are:

- the inactivation of a free radical within the cell just after its creation
- the mopping-up of free radicals by scavenging antioxidants

- the increased elimination of material already damaged by free radicals

Returning to the party analogy, trouble would be prevented if the single man was not there in the first place, and similarly we can avoid exposure to free radicals from such sources as pollution, bad diet, and smoking. His being stopped at the door could be likened to free radical inactivation and if he was picked up inside the room by a wandering bouncer we could compare that with free radical scavenging. If, as soon as he finds his woman, he is escorted out of the party immediately we have the analogy with the elimination of already damaged material. So, you see that there are several stages which lead to complete free radical mayhem, but potential problems can be prevented at each one of these different levels.

Examples of some of the antioxidants, or free radical fighters, in your body are the vitamins A, C, E, the mineral selenium, and such chemicals as catalase, idebenone, superoxide dismutase (SOD) and glutathione. But there are hundreds of others.

One part of the cell which is most susceptible to free radical damage is its outside shell, i.e. the cell membrane. The cell membrane is composed mainly of lipids (fat) and proteins. The lipids on the membrane are very liable to interact with free radicals and produce a chemical called malondialdehyde (MDA) which we will be referring to later on in the book. MDA is a dangerous byproduct of free radical activity and can cause further harm to your tissues. There are many other byproducts of free radical damage, which not only cause further damage themselves, but also contribute to another important ageing process called glycation which I will discuss a little further on.

WHAT YOU CAN DO TO REDUCE FREE RADICAL INJURY

Oxidation is the price you pay for breathing oxygen. Oxidation creates free radicals which contribute to ageing. You can limit your exposure to free radicals in a variety of ways: I have already mentioned avoiding smoking, pollution and a bad diet, all of which can increase the production of free radicals and deplete your body of antioxidants. Everyone knows the benefits of a healthy, active lifestyle and I do not need to discuss these here.

Another way of limiting free radical hits is to take more antioxidants, both in the diet and by supplementation. There are people who say that it is not necessary to use supplements, and that humans have managed to survive for thousands of years without taking antioxidant tablets. The problem is, however, that we now live in a technological era which, for the first time in human history, increases our exposure to free radicals through artificial radiation, the depletion of the ozone layer, pollution with chemicals in every part of the 'civilized' world, stress, hormone-treated animals and toxins in foods.

Under these circumstances, it is not unreasonable to assume that you might need to supplement your intake of dietary antioxidants with additional supplements in tablet form, in order to counteract all the hostile aspects of our modern environment.

Examples of common antioxidants, apart from those which I have already mentioned are:

- pycnogenol
- lutein
- co-enzyme Q10
- isoflavones in general

These and many others are found in plant chemicals (phytochemicals) as well as in fish and animal products. Consuming a diet rich in fruit, dark-coloured vegetables, fish and lean meat can go some way to providing your body with certain necessary antioxidants, but you also need to take supplements for the reasons I have already given. I will be discussing several of these supplements in more depth later on in the book. Some of the natural antioxidants not only fight free radicals but can also take part in other processes such as glycation. Carnosine is a typical example of an antioxidant which is also an anti-glycation nutrient.

GLYCATION

Before I move on to another age-related process, that of glycation, let me briefly explain what a protein is. Proteins are valuable biological molecules which play a huge part in maintaining normal life. They are found in almost every part of the body and have a variety of functions. For example, proteins are present inside the cells, carrying oxygen and other nutrients to the tissues and making the life of the cell possible. They are also present outside the cell as parts of the immune system fighting bacteria and viruses.

Proteins are formed by long strings of amino acids. These are relatively simple chemicals – lysine, methionine, and arginine, to mention a few. If you imagine a protein as a wall, amino acids are the individual bricks. However, proteins are not straight lines of amino acid sequences, but have a certain normal configuration.

For example, in a three-dimensional world, a particular protein may go five amino acids straight up, six amino acids to the left and down, three towards you, five to the right and up, and so on, making it a complex structure like a very twisted stick. Any change to this configuration and the protein loses its normal function. You will see why this normal protein configuration is so relevant when I discuss glycation.

The process of glycation (also called glycosylation) is turning out to be almost as important as oxidation in causing age-related damage. Glycation happens when glucose molecules (and other sugars such as fructose, or other similar chemicals such as aldehydes) attach themselves to proteins. MDA (malondialdehyde) is an aldehyde which is very keen to take part in this reaction. Other aldehydes which can also take part in glycation are acetaldehyde and the more familiar formaldehyde. This attachment of sugars to proteins is responsible for causing a brownish discoloration of tissues. This is not as innocent as it might sound. Why? Because this combination of sugars and proteins (i.e. glycation) causes proteins to bind to each other. Let me explain why this matters.

Normally, proteins are not supposed to be bound to one another. There are exceptions, of course, but let us concentrate for a moment on this rule:

- protein does not, and should not attach to another protein
- protein can attach to sugar
- sugar can attach to protein

Therefore, the end result of this is that a protein which is attached to a sugar is liable to interact with, and bind to, another protein. This is called 'cross-linking' and is not good news at all.

Imagine your hands are two individual proteins. They are free to do what they like, when they like, independent of each other. They are there to serve you and protect you. Move them around. They are not bound together. Bring your thumbs together and try to keep them attached to each other. Nothing happens. Your hands are still free to move around. Now imagine putting a good amount of extra strong glue – the equivalent of a sugar molecule – on one thumb – the equivalent of a part of the protein. Bring your thumbs together again. You will see that your thumbs now bind firmly together, making your hands unable to move independently and unable to do anything useful. This is 'cross-linking' in all its glory.

A cross-linked protein is not only useless but can cause more damage by reacting with free radicals and other toxins to create grotesque biological material called advanced glycation end-products (AGEs). These are the equivalent of what happens when your thumbs are cross-linked, i.e. when they are glued and bound together. You will start dropping things on the floor, spilling your drink, making a mess, all of which makes life more difficult.

Just as with the free radicals and the party analogy mentioned above, there are several intermediary stages during the process of glycation. These stages, with their 'thumb' analogies are:

Stage 1. The approach of a sugar/aldehyde molecule to the protein – getting the glue ready

Stage 2. The actual attachment of the sugar/aldehyde molecule to the protein and the creation of an activated protein, ready to be cross-linked – applying glue on the thumb. This particular step is called 'carbonylation', see below.

Stage 3. The cross-linking of the proteins – the binding together of the two thumbs

Stage 4. The formation of AGEs – the combination of the two disabled thumbs and the damage they cause as a result.

Also, as with the free radicals and the party analogy, there are different steps where glycation can be blocked. Referring to the above four stages, here is a possible plan of action:

Protection step 1. Avoid exposure to glycating agents by avoiding a high carbohydrate diet – or block these as soon as they are formed – inactivate MDA for example

Protection step 2. Immediately cover or protect the carbonylated protein – for example, by using carnosine, as will be explained below

Protection step 3. Break the bond between these proteins, or get rid of those proteins which are already cross-linked

Protection step 4. Fight AGEs and related damage with antioxidants and with other anti-ageing drugs.

The reason why AGEs are called 'advanced' glycation endproducts, is simply because they are the end result of an advanced stage of the glycation process (stage 4). These monstrosities are real troublemakers, circulating in the body and causing a lot of harm, contributing heavily to what we call 'ageing'. AGEs cause further cell damage when they attach themselves to the cells, at special attachment sites called RAGEs (receptors for AGEs). When they bind to the cells they stimulate the production of several poisonous chemicals within the cell. The end result is destruction of the cell, plus creation of further toxic by-products (MDA for example) which start all over again in a vicious circle.

AGES are found in most tissues of your body, and their concentration increases constantly from the age of twenty onwards. A large amount of AGEs in the brain has been blamed for contributing to Alzheimer's dementia, because AGEs increase the formation of amyloid beta. This is a toxic material found in the brains of older people and it is particularly abundant in Alzheimer's dementia patients. Apart from amyloid beta, AGEs also stimulate the production of other dangerous compounds such as certain free radicals (including nitric oxide or NO) and others such as interleukin-6 and tumour necrosis factor. I will explain more about these toxic, inflammatory compounds later on.

Let me return to the details of cross-linking. I have explained how 'bad' chemicals such as aldehydes and sugar derivatives, can bind to proteins and 'turn them bad'. This particular step in the process of glycation (stage 2 in the above example) is so important means that the sugar compounds add chemicals called 'carbonyl groups' to the protein in preparation for a full cross-linking.

Ageing is associated with an increased number of carbonyl groups on proteins which is a way of saying that during life many of our proteins get earmarked for destruction and can do little else but get cross-linked. About a third of all human proteins become carbonylated in later life. A carbonylated protein is like a thumb with glue on it, ready to be cross-linked at any moment.

I mention all of these apparently complicated steps for a reason. As you will see later in the book, cutting-edge research shows that the nutrient carnosine can block these carbonylated proteins and inactivate them, preventing them from being cross-linked. Returning to the analogy of the glue on your thumb, if you stick a piece of paper on your glued thumb before you touch the other thumb, then your thumbs may look a mess but they will not attach to each other, leaving you free to move your hands. Here, carnosine is the equivalent of the piece of paper. A protein which has been protected by carnosine is said to be 'carnosinylated'. This is a protective benefit of carnosine which tries to patch up carbonylated proteins before they attach to other proteins.

So, to summarize:

- A protein with a carbonyl group on it is called 'carbonylated' – glue on thumb.
- A carbonylated protein which has reacted with carnosine is called 'carnosinylated' – piece of paper on the thumb with the glue.
- A carbonylated protein which does not have the benefit of carnosine protection and has been allowed to react with another protein is called 'cross-linked' – two thumbs glued together.

As mentioned above, MDA is a real troublemaker – the equivalent of the glue – attaching itself to healthy proteins and making them liable to be cross-linked. Where does it come from? It is the result of free radical damage to lipids (fatty constituents of cells). You see now how oxidation and glycation are linked. Oxidation creates free radicals which produce MDA which causes glycation which results in AGEs which create more free radicals which produce MDA which... and so on, until you die.

However, all is not lost. There is hope, in the guise of the nutrients such as carnosine and other anti-ageing drugs. These can break this cycle because they interfere with MDA. They do this in the following ways:

A. Combining with MDA and inactivating it before it can cause any damage (the equivalent of prevention step 1 above). This is how lipofuscin is formed. Lipofuscin is a relatively inert material found in increased amounts in your tissues during ageing, manifesting as brown skin spots for example.

B. Repairing proteins already damaged by MDA, those carbonylated proteins which, although not cross-linked yet, are ready to be cross-linked in a short time (the equivalent of prevention step 2 above). The carbonyl group is covered and inactivated by certain anti-ageing drugs so the protein cannot cause any more harm through being cross-linked. These proteins are then eliminated in several stages and taken out of the system (part of prevention step 3 above).

Ordinary antioxidants such as vitamins E and C are active against free radicals but they do not do anything against glycation. However, newer anti-ageing agents such as carnosine and metformin are active both against free radicals and against glycation. One reason why these agents are effective against glycation is because their chemical structure is similar to that of other chemicals which cause glycation, and they can therefore easily attach themselves onto the protein, protecting it against any intruders.

Examples of clinical impairment resulting from glycation are:

- The wall of the arteries becomes thick and inflexible and crumbles easily, resulting in high blood pressure, heart attack or stroke.
- The inside of the brain cells gets clogged with abnormal biological material (amyloid beta) resulting in loss of memory and contributing to dementia.
- The skin proteins and collagen clump together, and then collapse to form wrinkles and grooves on the skin.

Unfortunately, the process of glycation not only affects proteins but also interferes with the DNA. For example, sugar molecules can cause abnormal bonding between a DNA molecule and a protein, also by cross-linking. A cross-linked DNA molecule is of no use at all. The trouble with glycation was always thought to be that the bonds it forms are permanent. When two proteins (or a protein and a DNA molecule) are cross-linked, it was forever. We can prevent cross-linking but we could not break the abnormal bonds formed between two already cross-linked molecules. This is very important because it illustrated the irreversibility of ageing. When the damage had already been done we could do nothing to reverse it. If we were able not only to prevent, but also to reverse cross-linking, if we could break the bonds already formed between two proteins, then in effect we would be reversing ageing, making the proteins 'young' again (the equivalent of prevention step 3 above).

Until now, breaking existing bonds between already cross-linked proteins *was* thought to be impossible. Not any more. Later on I will discuss further a new, state-of-the-art group of drugs (for example, one called ALT711) which can actually break existing bonds between proteins, which is the equivalent of applying special solvent to two glued thumbs, dissolving the bond and freeing the hands again. This shows that ageing is not completely irreversible. Let me now move on to another important age-related process, that of methylation.

METHYLATION

During methylation, chemicals called 'methyl groups' are being added to different constituents of the proteins, DNA and other molecules to keep them in good, active condition. Examples of useful chemicals which need to be methylated are:

- the antidepressant, 'feel-good' brain chemical, serotonin
- the useful stimulant hormone, adrenaline
- the 'good' fat molecules, HDL
- certain constituents of the cell membrane called phospholipids (including the chemical phosphatidylcholine).

Without methylation, none of the above chemicals would be able to stay around for long. Generally speaking, methylation is necessary for the normal maintenance of your tissues, and it is usually kept at healthy levels naturally by your body. However, like most processes related to ageing, things are not that simple. While moderate methylation is good, excessive and unbalanced methylation is not something you would want. I will explain why, shortly.

A good aspect of methylation is that methyl groups move around the blood stream, piggybacking on special chemicals. These carrier chemicals are called 'methyl donors' because they donate their extra methyl groups to any other molecules that need to be methylated. One of these methyl donors is called SAMe (S-Adenosyl-Methionine) which is one of the most important methylators in the body. Another methyl donor is TMG (trimethyl-glycine), which, as the name suggests, carries three methyl groups. It is a kind of molecular camel, laden with its cargo of methyl groups. I will refer more to these two friendly compounds later.

A few examples of situations where methylation is essential are:

1. A methylation process transforms the nutrient carnosine into its cousin called 'anserine' which is a more stable and not so easily destroyed compound.

2. Methylation of certain parts of your DNA causes the permanent switching off of unnecessary genes and saves your body from abnormal DNA division.

This means that methylation of those particular sections of DNA blocks any abnormal DNA from being passed on to future generations of cells.

3. Methylation of the dangerous chemical homocysteine transforms it into the harmless amino acid methionine.

4. The amino acid arginine needs to be methylated to its sister molecule called 'mono-methyl-arginine' which is a really useful compound to have in the brain. It adjusts certain brain receptors (binding sites), particularly the NMDA receptor which plays a part in inflammation and excitotoxicity, two age-related processes, which will be briefly discussed later in the book.

The problem is that methylation can plummet during certain stages of life. For example, any chronic inflammation process can affect methylation because the immune system, which is heavily involved in fighting inflammation, gorges itself on methyl groups, leaving nothing for other tissues of the body. From this example you can see the overlap of two theories of ageing, the theory of methylation and that of inflammation. One process can affect the other, and fighting one aspect of ageing may have a repercussion on other parts.

Low methylation is reflected in the increasing levels of the nasty chemical homocysteine, which is found in chronic inflammation processes such as lupus, heart disease and diabetes. An increased intake of methylators has been shown to reduce the risk of these diseases. Heavy exercise also increases the demand for methylating chemicals to fuel the muscles during exercise, so methylation for the rest of the body takes second place, and becomes neglected. The moral of this? Do not exercise excessively.

UNBALANCED METHYLATION

The bad news is that methylation is not completely foolproof. Yes, it is useful for some body parts, but if left unbalanced it can deregulate other parts. It can, for example, switch off useful genes which protect you against cancer, or it can activate other genes which promote cancer. The methylation process becomes relatively unbalanced during ageing, resulting in DNA, collagen and protein destruction, as well as interfering with several normal reactions which are thirsty for methyl groups.

Everything involved in ageing is a matter of balance. Too much is bad. Too little is also bad. Some methylation is essential, and any age-related loss of methylation increases the rate of cell death. Free radicals add insult to injury in this respect by speeding up the destruction already caused by defective methylation. On the other hand, certain parts of the DNA, if excessively methylated, may also cause damage or even cancer.

Are there any practical steps you can take to help yourself? Your body is usually a good judge regarding which parts need methylating and which parts do not. So if you try to keep a good level of methylating nutrients in your diet and take methylating supplements, as discussed later, your body will then decide how best to use these for its own benefit.

OTHER PROCESSES INVOLVED IN AGEING

Apart from the trio of oxidation, glycation and methylation, there are two other main processes which are implicated in nature's devilish plot to age you. One is chronic inflammation and the other is hormonal deregulation. Let us deal with inflammation first.

There are scientists who believe that most age-related changes in the body are due to chronic inflammation. When there is chronic inflammation the body tissues are eaten away by toxic chemicals, resulting in dementia, thickening of the arteries, arthritis, diabetes, hormonal imbalance and so on.

A particular component of chronic inflammation is excitotoxicity This happens when the brain cells are overexcited. The brain chemical, glutamate, is normally responsible for stimulating the different parts of the brain, but too much glutamate results in overexcitation and the eventual death of the cell. The results of excitotoxicity are seen in strokes and Alzheimer's dementia. As I shall explain, carnosine protects against excessive glutamate activity, and thus reduces excitotoxicity.

The chemical MDA has also been implicated in inflammation – as if its behaviour in causing glycation was not enough – and so any drugs which inactivate MDA have anti-inflammatory benefits. Chronic inflammation has been associated with a chemical called tumour necrosis factor (TNF) which is found to be high in Alzheimer's disease and in multiple sclerosis, to give two examples. TNF actively promotes degeneration of your brain and nerves. It is activated by a combination of AGEs and free radicals, and needs to be kept as low as possible. There are several agents which reduce TNF – for example adaptogens and calorie restriction mimetics, both of which we will discuss at greater length later.

Chronic inflammation and brain damage can also be caused by a dangerous by-product of nitric oxide (NO), called peroxynitrite. This is the result of the oxidation of NO, and it is a major toxic by-product. It can, for example, worsen atherosclerosis. Antioxidants (such as co-enzyme Q10) may help foil the actions of peroxynitrite.

A handful of doctors suggest that people should be using low doses of anti-inflammatory chemicals such as aspirin, ibuprofen or diclofenac to keep age-related inflammation at bay. This is not a widely shared opinion however. A diet containing nutrients which can reduce some of the effects of inflammation is, however, a good idea. Such a diet should include fish (which contains anti-inflammatory oils), fruit and vegetables (particularly berries which are packed full of antioxidants and inflammation-fighting flavonoids) and supplements of alpha lipoic acid which is a well-known inflammation fighter.

HORMONES

Now we come to the fifth and final major process involved in ageing, and that is hormonal deregulation. This theory says that ageing results in a general hormonal imbalance within the body. In plain terms, your hormones go haywire with the passage of time.

Drs Dillman and Dean explained the effects of this hormonal imbalance, and if you are interested in exploring this further, you need to read their book *The Neuroendocrine Theory of Ageing and Degenerative Disease* (The Center for Biogerontology, Pensacola, Florida 1992). What has relevance here is that hormones such as growth hormone, melatonin and DHEA need to be replaced or reactivated during ageing to prevent your body from falling apart. Not only that, but the binding sites, where the hormones attach themselves onto the cells need to be in good working order, otherwise the hormones will be unable to operate properly.

Some scientists, however, flash a warning. Your supplies of growth hormone or DHEA may well dry up as you grow older, but perhaps this reduction is not a dangerous thing after all, and may happen for a reason. It may, for example, prepare your body to become better able to cope with the changes of increasing age. Those who gorge themselves on extra supplements of hormones may be interfering with a natural defensive mechanism, throwing a spanner in the normal workings of hormonal balance. Some scientists even say that growth hormone replacement may accelerate ageing, in the long term.

This is one point of view. Many anti-ageing doctors, though, believe the opposite is true. They believe that if the level of something is high in youth and low in old age, then replacing that something should make the physical aspects of youth reappear.

So, these are the main processes of ageing and I trust that this discussion of them opens up some opportunities for action which may protect you against the devastation ageing can cause. Many people ask me whether ageing can be reversed. My answer is that it depends on what you mean by 'ageing'. Commonly available products cannot reverse all aspects of ageing as a whole. They may be effective on a single age-related process such as oxidation, glycation, methylation, or inflammation, but they are not able to influence the entire ageing process. Academics and laboratory researchers believe that the word 'ageing' has scholarly and scientific connotations such as 'an increased force of mortality', 'cellular senescence', 'replication arrest' or 'action of pleiotropic genes'. Others believe that ageing means something more tangible – such as grey hair, loss of memory, wrinkles, arthritis, osteoporosis and so on. According to this view, which is the one I take in this book, it is indeed possible to prevent and reverse ageing.

Anti-ageing medicine uses products or procedures which claim to be able to:

A. *Protect* against certain aspects of ageing such as oxidation, glycation or inflammation. These include products such as carnosine, adaptogens, co-enzyme Q10 and antioxidants, which may deal with only one or two of the mechanisms of ageing.

B. *Reverse* a. the clinical signs of ageing through the use of DHEA, growth hormone, face lifts and skin products, for example. These can change the way you look but they do not affect your rate of biological ageing. b. actual biological ageing through the use of ALT711, telomerase or cloning. Such methods have been shown actually to reverse biological ageing and turn back the clock in a limited way, on a handful of occasions.

You will see from what I have said that the 'elixirs of youth' I discuss have good points and bad points. Some of them are not so well studied, whereas others are studied but with negative results. The benefits and drawbacks of all the remedies discussed in this book will be highlighted. So without further ado, let us start with the first serious anti-ageing product, carnosine.

CHAPTER 1

Carnosine

WHAT IS CARNOSINE?

Carnosine is a combination of the amino acids b-alanine and L-histidine. Some people confuse carnosine with another chemical called 'carnitine'. This, however, has nothing to do with carnosine and it just happens that these two have similar-sounding names. The same is true for other variants of these two compounds. For example, I will refer later to acetyl-carnosine which has nothing to do with acetyl-carnitine.

Carnosine is found in massive quantities in muscle, including the heart muscle, where it is one of the most abundant chemical compounds, and in the brain, particularly in the olfactory nerve, which is responsible for the sense of smell. Smaller quantities are also present in the kidneys and in the stomach. Examples of carnosine-rich foods are chicken breast, rabbit leg, frog, sturgeon, beef leg, and duck and turkey meat.

The overall concentration of carnosine in both animal and human tissues dwindles with age. For example, in some instances the carnosine levels may plummet by 10% every 10 years. This lack of carnosine may be due to the loss of muscle tissue which is a common legacy of increasing age. Less muscle tissue means less carnosine.

There are several similar variants of carnosine, and the following are examples:

- anserine (produced by methylation of carnosine)
- homocarnosine
- N-acetyl-carnosine (also called N-alpha-acetylcarnosine)
- carcinine

There is a serious effort by commercial manufacturers to make some of these variants available in capsule form for the general public. However, apart from carnosine, no other variants have been shown to have clear benefits when taken orally. acetyl-carnosine is quite effective if it is used in eyedrops.

CARNOSINASE

This is an enzyme which breaks carnosine down to its individual constituents – histidine and alanine. While some people believe that carnosinase is harmful, because it destroys carnosine, others are not so sure. The breaking down of carnosine to histidine and alanine may be a valuable natural source of these two amino acids. Alanine, for example, is needed during processes which stimulate the formation of new genetic material and new collagen, whereas histidine fights muscle fatigue and stabilizes the inflammation reactions following an allergy. It can also reduce the severity of breathing difficulties experienced by some athletes after strenuous exertion. Let us look at these individual components of carnosine in more detail.

ALANINE

Alanine on its own (i.e. when it is not incorporated onto the carnosine structure) is an important amino acid found in muscle tissue. It is obtained from beef and pork, oats and wheatgerm, and cheese, yoghurt and other dairy products. Sometimes alanine supplements are used by diabetics who want to reduce the high amount of sugar in their blood. Alanine can also stimulate certain special immune cells, the leukocytes, and can therefore benefit people who have a weak immunity. It is present in the prostatic fluid – the fluid produced by the prostate to lubricate the sperm – and some men are now using alanine to boost the health of their prostate. At least one scientific study has revealed that taking alanine supplements can limit the symptoms of benign prostatic enlargement. No side effects or interactions have been reported.

HISTIDINE

If you consume enough meat, poultry, fish, wheat, rice and rye, you should be getting sufficient supplies of histidine. This amino acid is invaluable during normal growth and repair in the body. It preserves the protective myelin sheath around the nerves, flushes out toxic metals from the body and balances the stomach fluids. People with rheumatoid arthritis frequently have reduced reserves of histidine, and so they take extra histidine supplements for its possible benefits. Many histidine users report improved sexual arousal and better enjoyment of sex. High amounts of histidine in the diet increase the levels of carnosine itself in the tissues. Histidine-related compounds, including carnosine, are generally good antioxidants and regulate the normal death and replacement of cells, which brings me to the process of apoptosis.

Normally, your cells wither and die in an orderly and controlled manner, during a natural process called 'apoptosis'. It is necessary for cells to die when they become damaged beyond repair, as this gives new healthy cells a chance to grow and replace the old and worn out ones. Apoptosis is a programmed cell death, a kind of weeding-out of weedy cells. A slow, constant rate of apoptosis is normal, but a speeded up rate is excessive and results in the loss of a large number of cells. For this reason, apoptosis needs to be regulated and allowed to tick over at a slow rate. Histidine, carnosine and similar compounds do exactly this: they regulate apoptosis and so suppress any excessive loss of cells.

One of the main functions of carnosine is to prevent free radical injury, particularly to the fatty components of the cell membrane. Carnosine is a cell membrane stabilizer and protector. Cells with a damaged outside membrane are like balloons with holes in them – useless. Carnosine not only protects the membrane surrounding the cell, but also shields the membrane surrounding the mitochondria. These are tiny organs present inside every cell and are responsible for producing energy from different chemicals. The fatty components of the membrane are keen to interact with free radicals during a process called lipid peroxidation. The resulting by-products of lipid peroxidation – one of which is MDA – end up causing all sorts of further mayhem.

One way carnosine is able to protect against this is by lending a hand to other antioxidants such as vitamin E and SOD (superoxide dismutase). The benefits are clearly seen when a mixture of several antioxidant vitamins is used. Carnosine is especially fond of vitamin E and works exceptionally well with it. The presence of one increases the efficiency of the other, because carnosine works better in water, whereas vitamin E works in fat, so in this way both watery and fatty tissues are reached.

GLYCATION AND CARNOSINE

As I have discussed previously, glycation is the process of forming damaging bonds between proteins and sugars. The result could be the creation of cross-linked proteins and AGEs. I have also discussed the fact that carnosine reacts with the carbonyl groups of the proteins, making them less liable to be cross-linked. Carnosine is powerful in fighting all the stages of glycation.

It is particularly keen to bind to the sites of proteins where sugar/aldehydes attach. When these sites are blocked, the sugar is unable to react with the protein, and so the protein remains unharmed.

Another way that carnosine works is that it fine-tunes a chemical called glutamate, or glutamic acid, in the brain. Normally, glutamate binds onto certain brain cell receptors called NMDA (N-methyl-D-aspartate). This stimulates the release of nitric oxide which, in low amounts, arouses the brain and improves memory. By improving the supply of glutamate carnosine maintains the health of the brain. Too much glutamate, on the other hand, overstimulates the NMDA receptor which causes overproduction of nitric oxide which, in turn, overexcites the brain. The whole process is made worse by free-floating zinc or copper metals. Carnosine, by binding to the zinc and copper metals, modulates the NMDA receptor and calms things down. Carnosine is a 'modulator', a word which is encountered frequently in anti-ageing research. A modulator is a sort of mediator which does two apparently simple things – it increases what is low, and it decreases what is high.

Carnosine and Inflammation

One of the causes of ageing is chronic inflammation, as explained in the previous chapter. Chronic inflammation can be fuelled by excessive production of nitric oxide (NO), and I have already explained how excessive NO production may worsen brain function. Because carnosine reduces or blocks any excessive activity of NO, it may offer protection not only against oxidation and glycation, but also against the other age-related mechanism, that of chronic inflammation.

AGES stimulate excessive production of NO and other toxic compounds, adding more poisonous ingredients to the already deadly soup of free radicals. By reducing AGEs, carnosine also lowers the production of these toxins. It will be obvious by now that all age-related processes are connected and depend on each other. When a protective agent such as carnosine acts in one area of ageing, this has repercussions further down the line, in other age-related processes.

RESEARCH SUPPORTING CARNOSINE

The number of experiments exploring the diverse actions of carnosine is growing by the day. A great number of these experiments concentrate on the anti-glycating merits of carnosine and continue to discover more about its exact benefits. For example, in a recent experiment using sugars – such as glucose, fructose and ribose – and also aldehydes, Alan Hipkiss and his team at the University of London have shown that carnosine can protect against the injury these caused on muscle tissue. The surprising thing is that they have also discovered that certain other amino acids, such as lysine and arginine, can protect against this type of injury too, but that their byproducts, created when the reaction is over, may, on occasions, cause cancer. However, the byproducts formed between the reaction of carnosine and sugars do not cause cancer. This shows us that there is still an enormous amount which needs to be learnt, not only about carnosine but also about any other nutrients which are claimed to have anti-ageing properties.

HUMAN CLINICAL TRIALS

After evaluating and digesting the enormous amount of promising scientific information about the effects of carnosine in animals,

I decided to start using carnosine for its anti-ageing value on humans. During the summer of 1999 I was the first clinical physician to use carnosine specifically for anti-ageing purposes on healthy human volunteers.

Since then I have been using various strengths of carnosine on many of my patients. Initial assessment of a small number of patients who took 50 mg–100 mg of carnosine a day showed that they experienced a variety of benefits. Some of their actual comments were:

- 'It improved my clarity of thought.'
- 'People mention how well I look, and my sleep pattern is now normal.'
- 'It has improved my well-being, and my joints are more agile.'
- 'There has been a visible improvement in muscle tone, and a reduction of nocturnal cramps.
- 'I have a heightened libido.'
- 'My sense of smell has improved.'

Although several other patients did not report any obvious immediate benefits, most of them were willing to continue taking carnosine for general anti-ageing protection. No one has reported any side effects, even those who have been taking carnosine daily for over five years. These initial comments were quite encouraging and this made me want to go further, so I decided to study the effects of carnosine on the human body in more detail.

As I have already mentioned, MDA (malondialdehyde) is a toxic by-product, produced when free radicals attack lipids (fat), such as those found on the cell membrane. MDA starts its ugly work as soon as it is created, working hard to cross-link as many proteins as it can, but it is eventually eliminated in the urine.

There are tests which measure the levels of MDA in the urine and give an indication of the degree of destruction already caused by free radicals. There are, of course, many other toxic by-products of free radical metabolism, but MDA is one of the most well studied. Several experiments done on animals show that carnosine inactivates and reduces the levels of this dangerous MDA. It is worth mentioning that the higher the amount of carnosine present, the lower the activity of the MDA, which is another way of saying that MDA and carnosine are extremely hostile to each other.

There is at least one home testing kit which measures urinary MDA. This is called the Vespro Free Radical Test (available from Vespro Ltd, see Useful Addresses). The patient collects some early morning urine, and mixes it with the special chemicals from the test kit. The results are then compared to a coloured chart. The colours correspond to four different values of MDA in the urine which, in turn, indicate four levels of free radical activity in the body, as follows:

- White corresponds to an extremely low MDA, showing an optimal level of free radicals working within the cells.
- Light pink corresponds to a low MDA level, and indicates a low free radical activity.
- Pink is for medium MDA levels, corresponding to medium free radical activity.
- Dark pink means high MDA levels and a high free radical activity.

Because carnosine is able to neutralize MDA and protect the body tissues from it, the Free Radical Test is an ideal means of finding out whether taking carnosine supplements has any impact on the MDA concentration in your urine. Taking carnosine should help reduce the levels of MDA in the body, and this should be shown in the urine.

A UNIQUE TRIAL

Based on this premise, I designed a clinical trial to research further. This is one of the first – perhaps *the* first – clinical trials to study the dosage and direct anti-ageing actions of carnosine on healthy humans. Because of this, I present all the details of the trial as they appeared in the official paperwork.

Does Oral Carnosine Supplementation Affect Urinary MDA?

AIM

To examine the effects of oral carnosine upon the concentration of urinary malondialdehyde (MDA), in everyday situations (i.e. outside laboratory conditions).

BACKGROUND

MDA is a product of lipid peroxidation which is also associated with age-related cross-linking of proteins and DNA. Carnosine is thought to:

1. Prevent lipid peroxidation and thus reduce MDA production

2. React with, and inactivate existing MDA and thus also reduce MDA levels

Theoretically, introduction or withdrawal of carnosine supplementation should have a reducing or an increasing effect, respectively, on urinary MDA levels. This would possibly be a dose-dependent process.

MATERIALS AND METHODS

Oral L-carnosine (obtained from IAS/Pro-Found Products) was given to 20 healthy volunteers in a variety of dosages. This supplementation took place in addition to the participants' usual drug/supplement intake, which remained constant throughout the duration of the trial. Morning urine was collected and tested by the participants using a colorimetric test kit which measures urinary MDA concentrations (Vespro Free Radical Test).

PATIENTS

Male and female volunteers aged 40–75 were studied as follows:

A. Individuals who already were on carnosine were tested (day 1, baseline) and then asked to stop taking carnosine for one week. This was followed by a second urine test (day 8) and the carnosine supplementation was resumed. A final test was performed on day 15.

B. Individuals who were not on carnosine were tested at day 1, at day 8 (after using carnosine for a week) and at day 15 (after stopping carnosine for a week).

C. Individuals on increasing doses of carnosine were tested as follows: day 1 (baseline), day 8 (after taking carnosine 50 mg a day for a week), day 15 (after carnosine 100 mg a day for a week), day 21 (after carnosine 200 mg a day for a week).

D. The difference between a 50 mg and a 1000 mg daily dose was tested as follows: day 1 (baseline, no carnosine), day 8 (carnosine 50 mg), day 15 (carnosine 1000 mg).

DETAILS

The urine testing was performed in a 'single-blind' fashion, with only the examiner knowing the significance of the different colours. This was done in order to avoid patient-effected bias. The existing colours on the testing cards were numbered 1–4, and made available to the participants without any further details on their significance.

The results of the study were presented at the 2nd Monte Carlo Anti-Aging Conference in June 2001, and details were made available on a number of internet sites. The study has been peer-reviewed, and formal publication will follow.

RESULTS

In some volunteers a dose of as low as 50 mg a day was shown to have a measurable effect on the urinary MDA, improving it from 'high' to 'medium', or even to 'low'. Stopping carnosine for a week worsened MDA in two people. Others who did not experience any effects on 50 mg a day, were able to see a reduction in their MDA after increasing the carnosine to 100 mg–200 mg a day. Increasing the dose further, to 500 mg or even 1000 mg a day (in a limited number of volunteers) did not have any further effect on MDA, i.e. it did not improve the beneficial results already experienced while on 100–200 mg a day.

This shows that it is not necessary to take high doses of carnosine to overcome its destruction by carnosinases, and even 50 mg a day is effective in some people, particularly perhaps in those who have a genetic predisposition to a low activity of carnosinase. Overall, the ideal dose was found to be around 100 mg to 150 mg a day. It is preferable to use coenzyme Q10 and vitamin E together with carnosine, as many volunteers who were taking these two supplements experienced a quicker improvement of their MDA levels. Those volunteers who exercised heavily showed the worst initial results, having an increased MDA which indicates an increased activity of free radicals during exercise.

Some other volunteers who took carnosine did not show any changes in their MDA, and this could be due to having an increased carnosinase activity which destroyed carnosine before it could have any effects.

However, these are very early stages and no firm conclusions can be made regarding this. More research is planned using higher doses of carnosine.

THE USE OF CARNOSINE FOR SPECIFIC ILLNESSES

Over the years carnosine has been used to treat different illnesses, from arthritis and high blood pressure to ulcers and inflammation. The following are examples of clinical conditions treated with carnosine.

ARTHRITIS AND BONE HEALTH

It was some pioneering Polish doctors who first used carnosine specifically for improving joint health, nearly 60 years ago. At that time, doctors recorded encouraging results, including improvement of the symptoms of rheumatoid arthritis. The treatment was given by injection (0.5 mg-1 mg every other day). These early studies also showed a clear improvement of components of the blood which are usually connected with inflammation (for example ESR, or the erythrocyte sedimentation rate, and eosinophilic cells). The carnosine treatment was particularly effective when combined with physiotherapy. These experiments were later confirmed by other researchers, who used high doses of carnosine.

More recently, Japanese researchers experimenting with carnosine-zinc combinations on post-menopausal women with rheumatoid arthritis, found that this treatment reduces the severity of the symptoms. Their research showed that the carnosine-zinc combination reduces pain and strengthens the bone structure in the wrists, probably by stimulating the bone-forming cells, called osteoblasts, to produce new and healthy bone tissue. These are promising results, but we are still some way from seeing carnosine taking its place among the conventional, run-of-the-mill anti-arthritic drugs.

HIGH BLOOD PRESSURE

During experiments with cats and dogs, carnosine given by injection over 15 days was able to lower blood pressure quite significantly. This was also shown to be the case by Russian scientists in a few unconfirmed trials in humans. The reason why carnosine has not become a popular treatment for high blood pressure is that there are other more potent drugs available. It is interesting to note that the drug ALT711, which will be discussed later on, is also thought to be able to reduce high blood pressure. Carnosine and ALT711 have similar actions, in that they both reduce the damage caused by glycation on the wall of the arteries, which then thickens the arteries and eventually results in high blood pressure.

In addition, carnosine has the extra bonus of being able to modulate NO (nitric oxide). Nitric oxide, in the right amounts, relaxes the arteries, thus reducing high blood pressure. Incidentally, NO also increases blood circulation to the penis. Indeed Viagra works by balancing NO, with the well-known uplifting results. Carnosine may also have a positive effect on erections, through its NO balancing acts, but this has not yet been studied in detail.

BLOOD CLOTTING

Platelets are small constituents of the blood which play an active part in blood clotting. If, for some reason, they clump together too much, they cause an excessive clotting of the blood, which may result in a blockage of the artery, manifesting as a stroke for example. If the platelets are a bit sluggish at clumping together, then the result is defective clotting of the blood with consequent haemorrhage. Carnosine has been shown to be able to modulate and regulate the action of platelets and in this way it balances blood clotting. In patients with abnormally quick clotting of the blood, carnosine decreases the clumping of the platelets, thus preventing stroke. In those patients who have an inability to control excessive bleeding, it does the opposite, stimulating the platelets to clump together and thus reduce bleeding.

ULCERS

Carnosine stimulates the formation of new skin (epithelium) over gastric ulcers, and stimulates other organs such as the liver and pancreas which, in turn, influence the workings of the stomach. Seeing an excellent opportunity, some entrepreneurial Japanese researchers have developed a carnosine-zinc combination with the brand name Polaprezinc. This is officially approved in Japan for the treatment of stomach and duodenal ulcers. When taken in tablet form, Polaprezinc remains inside the stomach for a relatively long time to cover the ulcer, after which the carnosine and the zinc dissolve and start healing the ulcer – simple and effective.

These researchers have shown that the carnosine-zinc compound reduces the damage caused by the bacterium helicobacter pylori on the stomach. Helicobacter pylori is a bacterium present in your stomach which, if allowed to multiply beyond a certain critical point, causes ulcers. The current conventional treatment for helicobacter pylori is with a combination of antibiotics and anti-acid drugs, but if carnosine is proven to reduce this bacterium in further trials it may well become a standard, worldwide treatment for ulcers. Polaprezinc is definitely a company to watch.

Polaprezinc has also been reported to be a strong anti-oxidant protecting the lining of the stomach. During an experiment performed at the Keio University in Tokyo it was shown that acid in the stomach causes extensive disruption of the DNA content of the stomach cells, but that Polaprezinc was able to reduce this.

WOUNDS AND SKIN HEALTH

It is a fact that applying carnosine directly on wounds speeds up the healing of the skin, without producing an exaggerated amount of collagen, which means that there is no excessive scarring. Brazilian and Japanese researchers have shown that carnosine speeds up production of granulation tissue, which is the healing material that fills a wound, just like cement fills in cracks in a wall. In another experiment, when carnosine was added to a nutritious formula given to people who had extensive wounds, it improved the rate of wound healing and it stimulated the natural mechanisms of repair.

Due to its anti-glycating properties, carnosine protects the collagen and elastin molecules in the skin. These are necessary molecules which give the skin its smooth, firm appearance. Other constituents of the skin – for example the fibroblasts and the material between the cells and the collagen which is called the 'extracellular matrix' – are also protected by carnosine. This is why Australians introduced carnosine cream for anti-ageing skin care. They market their products under the trade name Beta Alistine. Clinical trials with this particular form of carnosine are still necessary to prove its effectiveness.

AN UNUSUAL ANTI-INFLAMMATORY

I am always surprised by the different ways a remedy can be used. So I was intrigued to find out that carnosine can be used in toothpaste. If used in this form, it was found to be an effective treatment for inflammation of the gums. It suppresses an excessive immune reaction and stimulates a sluggish one, bringing the system back to normal equilibrium. It activates and protects immune cells (called B cells and T cells) which are necessary in controlling inflammation.

Another unusual way of using carnosine is by nasal spray. Carnosine has a particular affinity for the olfactory nerve and can easily go from the nose, via the smell nerve, straight into the brain, stimulating it and protecting it.

CANCER

High doses of carnosine (1000 mg–3000 mg in tablet form, daily) have been used by Russian doctors to treat inoperable tumours, and to protect against the effects of radiotherapy or chemotherapy. In experiments using such high doses in humans, carnosine showed both short-term and long-term improvements, such as protecting against an excessive lowering of valuable white blood cells, the concentration of which usually plummets during chemotherapy or radiotherapy. It also stabilized the cell membrane after it was damaged by radiation. Cancer cells increase sugar production because they need the chemical energy from the sugar in order to survive. Carnosine blocks this by reducing sugar availability, and therefore it has the potential to starve cancer cells to death, by blocking their energy supply.

INCREASED LIFESPAN

The results of an experiment showed that mice fed on high doses of carnosine live, on average, 20% longer than mice fed on ordinary food. In other similar experiments it was shown that the average lifespan increases and that an increased number of animals live to reach old age. However, the maximum lifespan is not affected. The maximum lifespan is the maximum number of years (or months, from the mice point of view) that can ever be achieved, whereas the average lifespan is the average length of time people (or mice) actually live.

In a combined Russian-British experiment, the following changes were observed in mice fed on carnosine:

- improved glossiness of their fur
- a better ability to heal skin ulcers
- an improved posture

After another series of experiments, Australian researchers led by Dr Robin Holliday from Sydney, reported that carnosine extends the lifespan of human cells in the laboratory. Human fibroblasts are special cells typically present in the skin and they play a part in creating new collagen molecules. When physiological (i.e. normal, not excessive) amounts of carnosine are added to a mixture of these cells in the laboratory they live for about 20% longer, which corresponds nicely with the mice experiments discussed above.

These cells also become able to divide more times than usual. Normally fibroblasts can divide around 50 times after which they become unable to divide any longer and so they die. This is called the Hayflick limit, after Leonard Hayflick who first described the phenomenon back in the early 60s. His theories suggest that it is impossible to overcome this limit and therefore we are restricted as to the amount of time we can live. During the Australian experiments, however, it was shown that this is not true, because fibroblasts treated with carnosine could divide an average of 60 times, and sometimes up to 70 times, well above the Hayflick limit.

Other experiments confirmed that, apart from having their Hayflick limit extended, carnosine-treated fibroblasts were able to live to over 400 days, instead of the normal 310. A different variant of these experiments showed that cells were able to keep on dividing to live for 413 days, whereas similar cells not treated with carnosine died after an average of 132 days.

All of these results were seen in cells treated with normal amounts of carnosine as low as those normally found in living muscle tissue (i.e. not excessively high). These experiments also show that normal amounts of carnosine are slightly better than marginally higher amounts. In technical terms, 20mM concentrations of carnosine extend cell divisions to a total of 70 cell doublings, whereas concentrations of 30mM can only extend the divisions up to 64 doublings.

Ageing goes hand in hand with telomere shortening. Telomeres are parts of the DNA molecule – at the end of the molecule – which are usually long, protecting the DNA against defects during replication (i.e. during the division of DNA to create two daughter molecules of DNA). With age, the telomeres become progressively shorter and thus less effective, until the DNA cannot function any longer, eventually destroying the cell. Free radicals and other toxins accelerate the shrinkage of telomeres. Once damaged, the telomeres are almost impossible to repair. It would make biological sense if antioxidants could effectively protect the telomeres from free radical damage before this happens. It turns out that only carnosine is capable of this protective action, out of all the other antioxidants tested so far.

It is worth reminding you that there is a difference between experiments in animals and those in humans, but the initial results on carnosine are very encouraging indeed. Carnosine is one of the most promising nutrients which may help people to achieve their maximum lifespan potential, and increase the percentage of people who become centenarians. Carnosine was discovered just over 100 years ago and by using it this may be an age that most people should aim to reach.

CLEAR VISION

I am now going to discuss what carnosine can do to your eyes. One of its most exciting properties is its ability to treat cataract. Cataract is a very common cause of blindness worldwide, affecting over 17 million people. This is over half of the world's blind population. 'Cataract' is Greek for 'waterfall', and this describes the difficulty for patients who see things as if they are behind a waterfall. The conventional treatment of cataract is by surgical removal of the affected lens followed by a transplant with a new, artificial one. Taking antioxidants has been advised by some doctors to try and prevent further impairment to the eye, but this does nothing to reverse an already existing cataract.

There are different types of cataract which affect different parts of the lens. The lens of the eye is formed by fibres – strings of proteins and other chemicals – which are transparent, allowing the light to reach the inside of the eye and create a visual image. Free radicals which are active within the lens destroy the fibres, initiating changes that lead to cataracts. For example, free radicals speed up the destruction of biological membranes and of certain valuable proteins inside the lens, called crystallins. Damaged crystallins do not allow much light to pass through and this results in poor vision.

Normally the crystallins and other components of the lens are protected against free radicals by a strong presence of antioxidants such as glutathione, which is a very effective free radical quencher, as well as vitamins A and E and carnosine. However, increasing age reduces these antioxidants in the lens leaving it without much protection. When this happens, damaged crystallins inside the lens accumulate and cause a 'clouding over' of the lens which leads to this state of affairs known as 'cataract'. This is where carnosine comes in. Normally carnosine is present inside the lens in large amounts, which means that it has a natural role to play in protecting against the progression of lens damage. When cataract develops carnosine becomes severely deficient in the lens. Some people believe that this means that, when carnosine is low in the lens, cataract becomes inescapable.

One way carnosine works is by removing the peroxide compounds which are the leftover toxic products following damage to the cell membrane. Carnosine, and its relative N-alpha-acetyl-carnosine, not only have antioxidant benefits of their own but also boost the action of other antioxidants in the lens such as that of glutathione.

Experiments with rabbits show that adding a carnosine preparation to the lens increases the carnosine content inside the lens, i.e. carnosine is able to reach the lens if given externally in eyedrops. Carnosine can delve deep into the lens and even reach parts of the lens which other antioxidants are unable to reach as, for example, in posterior subcapsular cataract. This has been debated by some scientists who think that the variant N-alpha-acetyl-carnosine is much more able to penetrate the lens than ordinary carnosine.

Apart from free radical protection of the lens, carnosine is also active against glycation. Glycation inside the lens causes abnormal bonds between proteins and sugar molecules, creating thick and twisted proteins which are not transparent. With time, more and more proteins accumulate, causing the characteristic clouding over of the lens and consequent loss of vision. Because carnosine is a strong anti-glycator, it has been used as a serious anti-cataract agent.

One of the things that speed up the formation of cataract is radiation, typically ultraviolet (UV) radiation from the sun, but perhaps also radiation from mobile telephones, computer screens and even television screens. In experiments with lens extracts in the laboratory, when the lens was exposed to bright light for long periods, the production of abnormal proteins was speeded up which caused the early changes typical of cataract. In animals exposure to strong sunlight was found to have similar results. UV radiation causes a lethal cocktail of free radicals with names like superoxide anion, hydroxyl radical, singlet oxygen and lipid peroxide. All of these destroy the constituents of the lens, as explained above, resulting in cataract.

With regards to injury caused by artificial radiation from mobile telephones, this is thought to play a role in accelerating cataract but there is no agreement between scientists as to whether this is a real or an insignificant risk. It may be best to be on the safe side, however, and to consider the use of a phone shield and antioxidants, including carnosine, for any eventuality.

It has to be said that cataract is a very complicated process involving many other mechanisms which have not been studied in detail. Free radicals, glycation and UV radiation, as well as several immune reactions play an important role in the formation of cataract, but there are other processes which need to be considered and clarified.

However, because carnosine is active against so many different processes, it is being used to deal with the problems caused by cataract. Several experiments with dogs suffering from age-related cataract have shown the positive effects of carnosine in improving the condition. Note that I said 'improving' and not merely 'preventing'. Improving means that the damage was already done and carnosine has repaired it, has reversed it. In these experiments with dogs, when treatment with carnosine eyedrops was continued for four months, the cataract improvement was sustained, i.e. there was no worsening of the condition.

In an experiment by Russian researchers in 1997 involving 109 human patients, carnosine eyedrops at a concentration of 5%, were also found to be effective in healing eye infections such as keratitis, and other eye conditions such as corneal erosions, corneal dystrophy and keratopathy, and corneal ulcers due to herpes, and bacterial infections. This is probably due to carnosine's ability to stimulate the repair processes inside the eye.

In another experiment, a carnosine derivative was found to be able to reduce intraocular pressure. High intraocular pressure (i.e. pressure of fluid inside the eye) is related to glaucoma, so in theory carnosine could help patients with this condition, although further research is needed here. The Pharmacological Committee of the Russian Ministry of Health has approved carnosine eyedrops for the treatment of medical eye conditions.

Carnosine as it stands may be unable to stay in the eye tissues for long because it is inactivated by carnosinase. For this reason, a stronger and more difficult to destroy form of carnosine has been developed called N-alpha-acetyl-carnosine (NACA). This is basically carnosine fortified with a special chemical group called acetyl. NACA is not as strong as carnosine when it comes to antioxidant action, but it lasts longer in the tissues.

During recent years, researchers have been able to show that NACA eyedrops reverse the symptoms of cataract in humans. This form of carnosine can remain in the lens for quite some time and therefore can exert its benefits over a long period. In a classic experiment, Russian and American scientists studied 49 people with an average age of 65 years, who had been diagnosed with age-related cataract. Half of the patients were treated with NACA eyedrops, and the other half were not treated, but only used for comparison purposes.

After six months of treatment, over 40% of the carnosinetreated patients experienced an improvement in the transmission of light through the lens, and almost 90% of these patients were found to experience up to 100% improvement of vision and sensitivity to glare. Sensitivity to glare increases with normal ageing, due to light being scattered by the non-transparent lens.

After 24 months of treatment these benefits were still continuing. In other words, as long as the treatment continued, the patients were protected against age-related cataract. The control patients (those who were not treated with carnosine), experienced a normal worsening of vision as would have been expected in anybody of that age. No significant side effects were reported in this study. The researchers concluded that the acetylated form of carnosine (N-alpha-acetyl-carnosine) is a suitable non-surgical treatment for age-related cataract.

The results of this experiment are far-reaching, suggesting that cataract could not only be prevented but also cured with simple eyedrops. The same researchers have found similar results in earlier experiments with rabbits, and their results on humans have also been replicated by Chinese researchers.

During a preliminary communication I had with Dr Aimin Wang of the Harbin Medical University in China, he explained his clinical trials which showed that carnosine cures age-related cataract. In two experiments in 1997 and 1999, he and his coworkers studied 96 patients, whose average age was 60 years, with age-related cataract. They used 1–2 drops of carnosine in each eye, 3–4 times a day for up to 6 months. They found that the carnosine-treated patients experienced an improvement of their condition at an amazing cure rate of 80–100%, with no side effects. This ties in with what the Russians have found in the experiments mentioned above. In another trial, Dr Wang studied 1000 patients with cataract and found similar benefits. His team also used carnosine drops in other eye conditions and found it to be effective in improving general eyesight, giving clear vision and brightening the eyes.

Following these pioneering experiments, carnosine eyedrops are now used commercially, as a treatment of cataract. Results of ongoing studies are awaited to confirm the benefits beyond doubt. There is a debate as to which form of carnosine is the best to use in cataract. Some researchers say that the NACA form is best because ordinary carnosine may be transformed into histamine in the eye and cause toxicity. The problem is that we still do not know whether histamine can cause toxicity in the eye tissues specifically. In other words, we do not know whether the actions of carnosine as described for other parts of the body, also hold true for the eye. Until the issue is clarified, it may be best to choose eyedrops in the NACA form in preference to ordinary carnosine. In addition, there is a debate concerning other ingredients of the NACA eyedrops. Dr Babizhayev, who performed the original research on cataracts, believes that adding vitamins and other chemicals together with NACA inactivates the mixture and makes the treatment less likely to succeed. (More details can be found at the web site www.nacetylcarnosine.com)

A CARNOSINE-RICH DIET

For those people who want to enjoy some of the benefits of carnosine without taking supplements in tablet form, it is possible to follow a diet rich in natural carnosine. Carnosine is found in red meat and chicken, particularly chicken breast. It is also present in eyes and nervous tissue, so those who, like the

Japanese, eat fish eyes may be getting a good share of carnosine.

Reasonable amounts of carnosine are also found in sprinting game such as rabbits and hares, and in other poultry such as pheasant. This corresponds with current nutritional advice which recommends choosing game meat as being healthier than hormonally treated pork or beef. About 100 gm of meat provides an average 100mg of carnosine. Carnosine is not found in any fruit or vegetables. This is not surprising as the prefix 'carn-' in carnosine, comes from the Latin meaning 'meat' or 'flesh'.

Who Should Consider Taking Carnosine?

Carnosine supplements are ideal for three things:

1. General anti-ageing protection. Out of the five main causes of ageing, carnosine deals with oxidation, glycation and chronic inflammation, as well as being a potential hormonal receptor regulator.

2. Prevention of diseases such as cataract, cancer, muscle weakness, heart disease, diabetes and dementia.

3. Specific treatment of existing conditions such as cataract, ulcers, and diabetic complications under medical supervision, in higher doses than usual.

DOSAGE

There has been a lot of speculation regarding the exact dose of carnosine. The Life Extension Foundation in the United States recommends an average of 1000 mg a day (500 mg–1500 mg) of carnosine in order to overcome the destruction by carnosinase and leave some carnosine free to work on the body. They extrapolated this dosage from the dosage of carnosine used in radiation protection experiments with mice.

During those experiments a maximum oral daily dose of carnosine of 500 mg per kg of body weight was used, which is the equivalent of 35000 mg a day for an average human. In some Russian experiments with cancer patients undergoing radiotherapy a dose of 3000 mg was used. This, however, was aimed at treating radiotherapy damage, and so the high dose has no bearing on an average healthy person, who just wants to get some protection against ageing processes. Questions remain as to whether such high doses are really necessary.

In rats, positive results were seen with doses of as little as 2 mg per kg of body weight, the equivalent of around 150 mg for an average human. No toxic side effects were seen even when the dose was increased to 500 mg per kg of body weight. Remember that these doses are for rats and not humans.

As I have already explained, during preliminary clinical trials I performed with carnosine, a dose of 100 mg–150 mg a day was sufficient to affect MDA levels and the argument for the need to flood the carnosinase system with carnosine does not appear valid. As little as 50 mg of carnosine a day may effect measurable changes in the body.

However, there are clinical trials in progress using high doses of carnosine, trying to establish whether the 1000 mg dose is better than the 100 mg one. At the moment, as things stand, I think that the arguments support the lower dose (50 mg–150 mg a day) but this may well change in favour of the higher dose (1000 mg) when results of ongoing experiments are released. It is best to take carnosine together with vitamin E and co-enzyme Q10 for ideal protection. Almost any other nutrient can also be taken with carnosine and no adverse effects have been reported of carnosine interacting with other drugs or nutrients.

SIDE EFFECTS

No side effects have been recorded, apart from rare muscular problems such as mild trembling, when using a very high dose of carnosine (1000 mg a day). One of the main problems frequently encountered by carnosine users is that it may not have obvious immediate benefits for everyone. It is necessary for carnosine to be used for years to gain sustained anti-ageing protection, and the results may not be evident in the short term.

OTHER ANTI-GLYCATORS

The normal ageing process causes loss of collagen and elastic fibres, by glycation, not only of the skin but also of the heart and arteries. Chemicals that prevent or reverse glycation are therefore thought to be important in reversing ageing changes. Carnosine is one of these chemicals, but there are several others.

ALT711

A company called Alteon Corporation in the United States is researching several anti-glycators. Their most important product is ALT711 (a thiazolium salt with the chemical name: 4,5 dimethyl-3-phenacyl-thiazolium chloride). This has been used in experiments to reverse problems such as thickening and loss of elasticity of the heart, and of the arteries, and it reduces blood pressure and improves circulation.

Experiments with dogs show that ALT711 reverses age-related stiffness of the arteries by 40%, and improves cardiac function. Carnosine and similar products prevent cross-linking, but ALT711 actually breaks the bonds between already cross-linked proteins, i.e. after cross-linking has already taken place. The action of ALT711 is definite proof that damage from at least one basic biological ageing process can indeed be reversed. There are other 'cross-link breakers' such as PTB (phenacyl-thiazolium bromide), similar to ALT711, but these are not as well studied as it is.

There is no clear evidence at present to show whether carnosine can indeed break existing bonds, just like ALT711. Some researchers believe that this is quite possible, perhaps due to the ability of carnosine to increase glutathione which interferes with a certain type of chemical bond (called S – S bonds) on the cross-linked proteins. Carnosine is able to remove already cross-linked proteins, however, and so it leaves the cells unobstructed to form new and healthy proteins.

To give you an analogy, think of a cross-linked protein as a house hit by a small bomb. ALT711 can repair the damage and make the house appear brand new again. Carnosine prevents the bomb from falling in the first place, plus it bulldozes any already damaged houses to the ground and clears the rubbish, leaving the place free for a new house to be built. Ideally, carnosine and ALT711 could, in theory, be taken together to complement each other's actions, but at the time of writing ALT711 is not yet available to the general public.

AMINOGUANIDINE

Also marketed as Pimagedine, this is a typical anti-glycator. It prevents cross-linking but does not affect bonds already formed between proteins. Its actions are somewhat similar to those of carnosine. For example, it can inactivate carbonyl groups on proteins and so reduce the risk of cross-linking. It also reduces toxic aldehydes and it is therefore effective during the early stages of glycation. One of its actions is to protect the kidneys against glycation, and human experiments show that aminoguanidine reduces the amount of useful protein lost in the urine.

Other potential benefits are seen in diabetes, where it helps stabilize the blood glucose, as well as reducing LDL cholesterol. It increases the collagen scaffolding within the arterial walls of older people by 30%, thus strengthening the arteries. Side effects are limited to mild nausea and headache. The hydrochloride form of aminoguanidine, although more expensive, is preferable to the bicarbonate form which is difficult for the body to assimilate. The suggested dose is 150 mg–450 mg a day, divided into two or three doses.

TENISLETAM

This drug was first used as an anti-anginal drug and then as a brain booster. It inhibits cross-linking and it has been found to have some positive results in Alzheimer's disease, by reducing the amount of dangerous beta amyloid in the brain. It works by blocking the sites where proteins can be cross-linked, and so it has an action similar to that of carnosine and aminoguanidine. The current consensus is that it does not break existing bonds like ALT711 does.

PYRIDOXAMINE

Pyridorin is the brand name of pyridoxamine, a derivative of vitamin B6 (pyridoxine). It is a potent inhibitor of cross-linking and an AGE preventor. It also has some anti-oxidation properties. It prevents free radical damage to sugar molecules, and so it prevents sugar molecules from being activated to initiate glycation.

Pyridoxamine inactivates carbonyl groups, just like the other compounds mentioned above, and it is particularly effective in the later stages of glycation. It could turn out to have clinical benefits in diabetes and atherosclerosis and is currently being evaluated by the manufacturers of Pyridorin, who are planning to license it as a drug, needing a doctor's prescription and not as a nutrient. This is because the manufacturers want to make sure that it has no toxic side effects, particularly if used in high doses.

CHAPTER 2

DHEA

Having discussed oxidation and glycation as major causes of ageing, now is the time to talk about the hormonal changes which affect the body during ageing. The first major hormone implicated in the ageing process is DHEA.

DHEA stands for De-Hydro-Epi-Androsterone, although it could easily stand for 'don't hasten early ageing'. It is a hormone produced by the adrenal glands (small organs snuggled up near the kidneys) and it is created by a chemical reaction involving the dreaded cholesterol molecule. Cholesterol is not always up to mischief, but can sometimes behave itself and be of some use to you. DHEA is an essential starting point for the production of other hormones such as oestrogen and progesterone (the 'female' hormones) and testosterone (the 'male' hormone). It circulates in the blood under the form of DHEA-Sulphate, which is inactive, and needs to be reactivated by the cells into DHEA proper before it can start its good deeds.

Like several other hormones, its production plunges significantly with the passage of time. This fall starts from one's early twenties and continues throughout middle age. In some instances its levels fall to a meagre 30% of the youthful levels, and this is just at the age of 40–50. As I mentioned at the beginning of this book, a fall of a particular hormone with age may not necessarily be a bad thing, it may just be the way Mother Nature prepares you to deal with the rigours of ageing. However, it is becoming increasingly clear that this may not be the case with DHEA. Falling DHEA levels are associated with a number of illnesses which are connected to ageing.

SCIENTIFIC TRIALS

Although anti-ageing treatment with DHEA has been around for many years, it gained some scientific acceptance only in 1995, when the New York Academy of Sciences published a prestigious book summarizing all the positive points of DHEA. There are over 2000 scientific studies (most on animals, some on humans) which show that it has a positive role to play in ageing.

For example, in a study performed at the University of California it was shown that taking 50 mg of DHEA every day for six months, pushes the DHEA levels in the blood right up to those of youth. Up to 84% of women and 67% of men who took part in this particular study reported that the treatment made them feel better, both physically and mentally. When the dose was increased to 100 mg a day, in men only, their muscle strength and muscle tissue improved considerably. At that dose, their insulin-like growth factor 1 (IGF1) levels were also improved. As I will discuss later, this IGF1 is an important hormone intermediary which is responsible for improving muscle tissue, reducing fat and boosting the immune system – a really useful hormone.

A particular form of DHEA called '7-keto DHEA' is believed to be more stable and about 2–3 times stronger than the real thing. The 7-keto variety does not easily convert to oestrogen or testosterone and so it may be useful to those who want to avoid the side effects related to these two hormones. 7-keto also has a more powerful beneficial effect on the immune system. Animal experiments with the 7-keto variety did not show any significant side effects even at doses equivalent to a whopping 140 times the normal dose for humans.

During a highly publicized recent experiment, French Professor E. Baulieu and co-workers studied 280 healthy older people aged 60–79. Half of these people were given 50mg of DHEA every day for a year, whereas the other half only took a placebo, or dummy pill. This clinical trial was therefore handled correctly in that it was a double blind, placebo-controlled study, which is the highest standard of respectable scientific research methods. These are the results in those patients who were treated with DHEA:

- there were no obvious harmful side effects
- the concentration of DHEA in the blood returned to younger (higher) levels

- a small increase in testosterone/oestrogen was noted, equivalent to the benefits of mild HRT
- the formation of new bone tissue increased in women over 70 years old
- there was a significant increase in libido in these women
- all the participants, but particularly the women, experienced an improved skin health, with skin thickness and hydration increasing, and age-pigments reducing.

This is a serious supporting scientific study, which should allay any fears about side effects or about DHEA not being active or useful. As mentioned previously, however, this treatment does not turn the ageing clock back, but merely improves the external and internal appearance of the user.

In an even more rigorous study, a double-blind, crossover, placebo-controlled clinical trial (see the glossary for an explanation of these terms) people aged 40–70 were given either 50mg of DHEA a day or a placebo. Over 80% of those who took the DHEA reported an improved quality of sleep, better mental and physical well-being and an improved ability to handle stress, compared to only 10% improvement reported by those who took dummy treatment.

Facts about DHEA

It increases antioxidant activity in rabbits and, possibly, in humans.

It activates osteoblasts, the bone-forming cells.

It protects against LDL (the 'bad' fat), particularly in older people and thus reduces the risk of heart disease.

SOME OTHER BENEFITS OF DHEA

IMMUNE BOOSTER

Several experiments show that DHEA is able to keep chronic inflammation under control. Chronic inflammation is thought to be involved in causing illnesses such as Alzheimer's disease, arthritis, brain failure, heart disease, and kidney disease. DHEA is found to help reduce the effects of chronic inflammation in a variety of ways. For example, it reduces interleukin 6 (IL6) which is a chemical frequently found in immune diseases such as rheumatoid arthritis. IL6 levels increase with age and measuring IL6 is, in fact, a guide as to how quickly the body ages. In double-blind cross-over studies, 50 mg of DHEA was found to reduce IL6 and improve the actions of natural killer cells which are essential in eliminating foreign viruses or bacteria. DHEA also encourages the production of interferon which is a substance needed for fighting several inflammatory disorders. Interferon is most notably used in some cases of multiple sclerosis.

On the other hand, studies have also highlighted the negative side of DHEA. For example it does nothing to boost the immune system against influenza in older people. Some believe that high doses of DHEA may actually worsen the risk of some cancers such as those of the prostate or the breast.

HORMONES

DHEA increases IGF1 (an intermediary of growth hormone) by about 10%. You can see how one hormone like DHEA can influence another apparently unrelated one – growth hormone. In this particular case, the end result may well turn out to be a lowering of the risk of osteoporosis, because IGF1 stimulates the activity of osteoblasts – cells which form new bone. DHEA is also used in slowing the progress of certain cancers (except those of the prostate and the breast), but that treatment is, of course, undertaken under strict medical supervision.

Thymus Health

A 46-year-old volunteer was given DHEA tablets daily for a month. These were taken in association with growth hormone injections. At the beginning of the experiment the thymus of the volunteer was measured and found to be reduced in size, as would be expected in a person of this age. At the end of the treatment the measurements were repeated and it was found that the thymus of the volunteer had grown to the levels one would expect to find in a 20-year-old. There was also a considerable improvement in the volunteer's immune function.

Note: The thymus is the organ responsible for modulating the immune system and its size reduces with age. A small thymus gland means a less efficient immune system and a higher risk of infection. The above experiment is the first proof that growth hormone and DHEA supplements can reverse the age-related shrinking of the thymus and improve the function of your immune system as a result.

As I have mentioned above, when DHEA is produced by your body, or when it is taken by mouth, it may change into different hormones such as oestrogens and androgens (male hormones). In a study performed at the Department of Psychology at Washington University in the United States, doctors gave 50 mg of DHEA to a group of menopausal women for four weeks. They then measured the levels of hormones in these women and found that oestrogens caused an improvement of mental well-being, boosting memory and cognition. However, the presence of androgens reduced this benefit. One reason why some experiments fail to find clear benefits with DHEA is because it can have different effects on different groups of people, depending on their sex, age, health and so on. This is another reason why it should be taken only under medical supervision.

BRAIN HEALTH

Some experts believe that damage to the nerves happens at a faster rate when DHEA levels are low. In experiments, adding DHEA to nerve cells in the laboratory can make them stronger and better able to withstand chemical and toxic assault. In mice DHEA treatment improves memory and helps them remember their way around a maze. American scientists tried a special variant of DHEA, called 'hydroxyl-epiandrosterone', on laboratory animals. They reported that it has powerful cytoprotective (cell-protecting) effects, suggesting that it may have therapeutic potential in various neurodegenerative conditions such as Alzheimer's disease.

DHEA levels are about 50% lower in the brain of Alzheimer's dementia patients compared to healthy people of a similar age, and so it is now being used in experiments with humans to determine whether it has any definite beneficial effects on dementia. DHEA protects brain cells against excitotoxicity and against the formation of beta amyloid which, as I have mentioned, is found in the brain of patients with Alzheimer's disease.

The way in which DHEA works on the brain has been further evaluated by Brazilian scientists from the

Department of Biochemistry at the University of Rio Grande. They found that DHEA modulates the release of neurotransmitters from the brain – particularly the release of glutamate which needs to be kept well balanced. Too much glutamate causes excitotoxicity, whereas too little causes memory problems.

There is serious debate regarding the possibility that DHEA may or may not be a treatment for Alzeimer's dementia. In one large study no such benefit was found, but when the results were re-evaluated by different scientists a different conclusion was reached. Many scientists agree that there is enough experimental evidence to show that DHEA *may* be an effective treatment for Alzeimers's dementia. What they do not always agree on is the fact that there is still not enough proof that DHEA is *definitely* effective as a treatment for the disease. Obviously research is still being carried out, but what is important is that there is optimism that DHEA has the potential to improve memory and lessen the risk of brain disease.

GENERAL BENEFITS

In a review study, low concentration of DHEA in elderly men was found to be associated with an increased risk of dying. Other properties of DHEA include its ability to reduce the appetite particularly for fats, to help people lose excess weight and to improve the tone of the skin. In fact, DHEA together with other hormones and antioxidants is now being used in cream form to help reduce the visible effects of skin ageing. The antioxidant effect of DHEA was highlighted in a very recent study which showed that it is particularly active in the bowel and the liver, protecting both organs against free radical attack.

DOSAGE

The best way to take DHEA is as tablets, in a micronized form so that the active ingredient is easily absorbed in the gut. DHEA in the sulphate form – a much cheaper form to produce than the micronized one – may not be that useful to the tissues because it is not easily assimilated within the body. It can be used in capsule or tablet form, in skin patches, and even under the tongue for easier absorption. The recommended dose for the micronized form is 25 mg–50 mg daily and for the 7-keto variety is 12.5 mg–25 mg daily.

Women should not use high doses of DHEA because they are able to metabolize, or make use of, any artificially taken DHEA much more easily than men. This means that when a woman takes DHEA, it is easily turned into the different intermediaries, including the male hormone testosterone which produces bad side effects. High levels of testosterone in women can cause acne, growth of hair on the face and deepening of the voice. Not an attractive possibility by anyone's standards. For fear of these side effects scientists recommend that women should use a reduced dose, perhaps 15 mg–25 mg a day, or use the 7-keto form which does not easily turn into testosterone.

Having said that, there are studies which examined such high doses of DHEA as an extravagant 1600 mg–2000 mg daily, and found that they improved muscle tissue and reduced body fat without any significant side effects. These high doses may be relevant for people who have specific diseases and are under expert medical supervision. There is no obvious reason why healthy people should take anywhere near those high amounts.

The long-term use of low strength hormones has been supported by some experts – even by those opposed to the general idea of anti-ageing medicine – as possibly an effective way of treating some of the signs of ageing.

SIDE EFFECTS

It has been estimated that the natural, youthful production of DHEA by the body averages 25 mg a day, and this has been used as a guideline for adjusting the dose in tablet form. Taking anything over 50 mg a day increases the risk of side effects. Menstrual bleeding may return in some post-menopausal women, but the bleeding is usually light. Also, taking continuous high doses may make the adrenal glands switch off and stop producing whatever small amounts of natural DHEA they are still capable of.

DHEA is a restricted substance and, in some countries, needs a doctor's prescription. Having said that, there are suppliers who make it available for personal use only in certain instances. Regulations change all the time and it is best to check with your doctor for your particular requirements. Currently, the use of DHEA in the UK is under the control of the Home Office.

A Double Warning

Some users have reported severe depression after taking even two or three doses of DHEA but, fortunately this improved after stopping the treatment. Changing from ordinary DHEA to the 7-keto form did not cause any further depression in these users.

Men with prostate problems should not take DHEA, or at least take it only under close medical supervision. This is because it may increase the prostatic specific antigen (PSA), which indicates an increased risk of prostate cancer.

I know of several people who take DHEA whenever they remember, or use it in high doses which cause side effects. Taking DHEA is a serious business and, legal regulations apart, its clinical effects need to be evaluated by a knowledgeable physician. The correct dose for each individual needs to be monitored with regular blood or saliva tests. Usually, it is not necessary to do a test before the treatment starts because it is almost certain that the levels will be below normal. Most people start taking the treatment and do a test about three to six weeks afterwards when the dose can be adjusted, depending on the result.

To summarize with regard to DHEA, it has quite strong advantages with regards to preventing some physical signs of ageing, but it may cause side effects, particularly at high doses. The scientific evidence supporting it is good and growing, but it must be taken under medical supervision.

MELATONIN

Some people also take melatonin supplements, either on its own or together with DHEA. Melatonin levels also decrease with age and taking it in supplement form is therefore thought to have an impact on age-related problems. A combination of melatonin and DHEA is believed to work more efficiently, improving the chances of fighting age-related changes.

Melatonin is widely used for jet lag and also to improve irregular sleep patterns, so it may be useful for older people who usually have disturbed sleep. It is also a restricted substance in the UK and in some other countries, but it can be obtained with a doctor's prescription.

The anti-ageing benefits of melatonin have only recently been studied in humans. The great majority of research has only been done on mice and on other laboratory animals. One of the main proponents of melatonin is the Italian Professor W. Pierpaoli. At an anti-ageing conference, we discussed his latest research, which shows that post-menopausal women treated with melatonin experience an improvement in their symptoms, together with an improvement of their thyroid levels. The thyroid hormones normally fall with age, and it appears that melatonin has at least a partial beneficial effect in reversing this situation.

I mention this to remind you that hormones work together, and any intake of one hormone may affect the performance of another. This is the basis of the hormonal deregulation theory of ageing which says that, with age, our glands become less able to produce and utilize hormones and, as a result, certain age-related conditions become more pronounced. To counteract this imbalance, and to help the hormones work together again, hormonal supplements and receptor re-sensitizers are used.

CHAPTER 3

Growth Hormone

Apart from DHEA, growth hormone is an important component in the anti-ageing process. Although these are two different hormones, their effects and benefits are sometimes similar or overlapping. Trying to explain the effects of growth hormone is bound to be slightly more difficult than discussing DHEA because growth hormone is connected to several other related chemicals, the action of which needs to be explored. Do not be put off by this. When you understand the basics of how growth hormone works, then its actions and possible benefits will become much clearer.

Human Growth Hormone (hGH or simply GH) is also called somatotropin, and it is produced by the pituitary gland in the brain. This gland is a pea-size organ which also produces several other hormones such as TSH (thyroid stimulating hormone), and sexual hormones which stimulate the production of oestrogen.

As its name suggests, GH is necessary for stimulating normal growth and development in children and for maintaining health in adults. GH is a kind of a 'general construction specialist', needed during everyday activities, such as helping to replace damaged proteins, rebuild cells, replace enzymes and chemical messengers. A lack of growth hormone in childhood can result in stunted growth, and one of the main uses of GH is in treating short stature in children.

THE POLITICS OF GH PRODUCTION

The pituitary gland which produces GH does not work independently, but is under the influence of other regulating hormones and factors, produced by other parts of the brain. For example, GH production is under the control of GHRH (Growth Hormone Releasing Hormone). This factor is produced by the hypothalamus, an important organ in the brain which regulates other glands, just like a central command office.

GHRH is, as the initials explain, a hormone which stimulates release of growth hormone. Another chemical, somatostatin, blocks the release of GH, so GHRH and somatostatin are in a constant tug of war, trying to keep GH at steady, normal levels.

Other hormones such as oestrogen and testosterone may influence the secretion of GH. In fact, as I have already mentioned, most, if not all, hormones in your body depend on each other and none work on their own. GH itself can interact with other hormones such as DHEA which is itself a GH stimulant. An increased production of GH helps normalize low thyroid hormonal levels. Melatonin is a possible releaser of GH, and it is possible that that is how melatonin increased thyroid hormone in Professor Pierpaoli's research mentioned in the previous chapter – by releasing GH which increased thyroid hormone. So you can see that hormones are like individual players in an orchestra, all working together to produce and maintain a masterpiece – you.

When the pituitary gland decides to release GH, it does so in short pulses and not all at once. For example, GH is released at the beginning of sleep. In a 24-hour period, young men experience four main pulses of GH release, whereas young women experience more than four. Exercise and nutrition affect the frequency of these bursts – a bout of physical exercise results in a burst of GH release.

Once released, GH does not do all the work itself but works through an active and strong intermediary. This is produced in the liver and is called Insulin Growth Factor 1 (IGF1, also called somatomedin). Measurement of IGF1 in the blood gives a good indication of what GH is up to.

Both GH and its active equivalent IGF1 need to bind to the cell receptors in order to activate the cell. When the quality and quantity of these cell receptors decreases (as in ageing for example), GH or IGF1 will not be able to bind on to the cells, so they will not have any appreciable effect. The binding of GH to a suitable cell receptor is like the use of a key in a custom-made lock. If the lock is damaged, you can have as many keys as you like, but they will not open that particular lock. This is why some scientists say that it is not just a matter of giving extra GH supplements but also a matter of somehow activating the receptors so that the whole system can work in harmony.

So, to summarize:

1. GHRH is produced by the hypothalamus and stimulates the production of GH from the pituitary gland.
2. GH increases IGF1 in the liver.
3. IGF1 binds to cell receptors and activates the cells to work properly.

Any disturbance of this process, at any stage and for whatever reason, causes the problems related to the lack of GH.

GROWTH HORMONE DEFICIENCY

A deficiency of GH in adults becomes more severe with age and this can occur from the age of 35–40. Normally, GH production peaks during adolescence and then starts to fall. A 60-year-old man may have only one quarter of the GH secretion of a 20-yearold. Older people also have less frequent bursts of GH release, and these bursts are not as powerful and last for a shorter time than those of younger people.

The lack of GH which comes with age is sometimes referred to as 'somatopause'. The most important consequences of low activity GH are:

What does it mean?

Soma=body, from the Greek

Somato-tropin-a hormone that 'turns' towards (i.e. supports) the body (GH)

Somato-stat-a hormone that 'stops' the effects on the body

Somato-a hormone that 'mediates' the effects on the body (IGF1)

Somato-a pause in the growth of the body

- a loss of muscle tissue and strength
- an increase of fat, particularly intra abdominal fat (i.e. fat tissues inside the abdomen)
- a thinning of the bones, which may result in, or contribute to, osteoporosis
- a worsening of glucose metabolism by a reduction in the responsiveness of cells to the actions of insulin, which is a hormone responsible for lowering blood glucose.

There are many other age-related changes attributed to dwindling GH activities:

- decreased energy
- a loss of libido and sexual function

- grey, fragile hair and damaged skin – e.g. wrinkles, due to the loss of collagen, the production of which is normally increased by GH; wound healing becoming slow and imperfect.
- a worsening of mental function, with loss of memory, motivation and concentration
- a reduction of the effectiveness of the immune system.

THE REPLACEMENT OF GROWTH HORMONE

It is a scientific fact that replacement therapy with GH can reverse some, if not all, of the above changes or problems. This has been shown to be true in a number of scientific experiments reported in peer-reviewed, prestigious medical journals such as *The New England Journal of Medicine.*

It is quite surprising to come across respected scientists who say that treatment with GH does not reverse the effects of ageing. It does. Older people lose muscle tissue just because they are getting old, but when they have suitable GH treatment their muscle tissue improves – perhaps not to where it was before, but it improves nevertheless. This is a reversal of an age-related change. It may not affect the underlying rate of ageing in that it will not reverse the rate of the biological ageing clock, nor will it slow it down, but it can give an 'aged' person some of the characteristics of a younger person, albeit temporarily.

The problem is that there are many unanswered questions. We do not know for how long GH can safely be taken; what the best way is to take it; how to decide who is suitable to have the treatment; what to do to reduce the cost of treatment and to reduce its side effects; and whether there are any hidden surprises after long-term treatment. Whatever the answers to these questions may turn out to be, the physiological benefits of GH treatment are now well recognized.

For example, GH makes muscle cells stronger and healthier by increasing their uptake of amino acids. This anabolic effect has raised a glimmer of hope in people who have muscle-wasting diseases, or other myopathies.

GH helps to restore the wall of the bowel to a more youthful state. The lining of the bowel wall progressively becomes thinner with age, causing problems with the normal absorption of food. GH helps prevent this problem by increasing the thickness of the bowel lining. It could be possible to involve carnosine in this as an intermediary. A carnosinezinc combination was shown to be effective in stimulating the production of IGF1 in the stomach and in the bowel. This increases the number of protective cells in the stomach, and so reduces the damage caused during ulcer formation.

According to supporters of GH treatment, almost all age-related devastation may be improved and repaired following GH replacement. People on GH treatment report sharper vision, better exercise capacity, lower blood pressure, improved memory and a robust libido. Their skin texture improves, and age-related thinning of the skin is reversed. Wound healing and immunity also improve, which is why GH is sometimes used in debilitated patients after surgery.

GH works together with such antioxidants as carnosine or Q10 to soak up free radicals. It creates special chemicals called 'protease inhibitors' which prevent free radicals from further attacking the cells. Even after free radical injury has occurred, GH provides the necessary stimulation for repairing the damaged parts of the cell.

Formal prescribing regulations do not approve the use of GH for anything other than the treatment of stunted stature in children or of those adults who have a definite deficiency of GH resulting in a specific disease. GH is not licensed for use in normal ageing, although the regulations are not clear. According to the exact interpretation of the regulation, all middle-aged and older adults have low levels of GH and IGF1, resulting in specific diseases irrespective of the fact that they are age-related diseases, so GH therapy should, in theory, be suitable for them.

ARTIFICIAL GROWTH HORMONE

Modern GH is made synthetically in the laboratory through genetic manipulation. Previously, good quality GH was obtained from the brains of cadavers which was fraught with dangers as it could transmit CJD (Creutzfeldt-Jakob Disease), the human equivalent of BSE or mad cow disease. So, in this respect, the natural form of GH is greatly inferior to a synthetic form.

One of the problems of synthetic GH is that it has to be given by injection. It is also a very expensive treatment. Some doctors also believe that any benefits gained from using injectable GH may decrease with time because too much artificial GH may actually interfere with the normal function of the cell receptors and, as a result, become unable to access the inside of the cell. So it is best to use low, near-physiological doses during treatment. 'Too much' is not necessarily 'better'.

A REGIME OF GROWTH HORMONE INJECTIONS

The injections need to be given daily – sometimes several times a day – following blood tests to evaluate IGF1. A dose of four to eight units a week is considered sufficiently low and free from significant side effects. The results may become apparent after six to ten months of treatment. Follow-up testing is necessary, to keep an eye on the level of IGF1, as well as on the PSA (prostate specific antigen) in men in order to monitor any possible adverse effects on the prostate.

Any side effects from this injection treatment depend on the dose used. Use a high dose of GH and you increase the risk of side effects. Lower the dose and the side effects become less noticeable. Common problems (when the dose is too high) are:

- carpal tunnel syndrome with increased tissue swelling which compresses the nerve at the wrist causing wrist pain
- an increased tendency to diabetes. Diabetic patients, in particular, should only use GH under expert medical supervision, if at all.
- gynecomastia (breast enlargement in males)
- fluid retention
- high blood pressure
- acromegaly (enlargement of the extremities)
- deepening of the voice

Recent experiments also suggest that increased GH may worsen the risk of cancer of the colon, and some doctors believe that high and prolonged use of GH may actually accelerate ageing. So, there you have it. It is all a question of balance.

SECRETAGOGUES

Fear of side effects, the enormous costs of treatment, and drug licensing regulations have directed interest to investigating other ways of boosting GH within the body without giving artificial growth hormone shots. It turns out that there are a multitude of substances, both synthetic and natural, which can stimulate the secretion of GH by the pituitary gland.

These substances are called GH secretagogues – a secretagogue being a substance that stimulates a gland to produce another substance. GH secretagogues, rightly or wrongly, are currently very fashionable in the field of anti-ageing therapy. There are new products being announced almost daily and it is extremely difficult to be sure which are effective and which are useless.

Theoretically, all of the benefits of injectable GH are also possible with GH secretagogues, although some people say that secretagogues are even better. Proponents of the use of secretagogues maintain that the pituitary is perfectly able to produce and secrete GH, but that it stops doing so because it receives conflicting orders from higher up in the brain – for example from the hypothalamus, which tells the pituitary what to do via the stimulating agent GHRH. For some reason GHRH fails with age and so it does not stimulate the pituitary to secrete GH. Secretagogues aim to remediate this by remotivating the different parts of the brain which are involved in GH production.

It is generally believed that endurance exercise is one of the best natural ways to increase GH production. However the effects of exercise on GH in older people have not been studied in detail. One particular study did not find any increase in GH or IGF1 after a six-month exercise programme in older people. So, in order to be on the safe side, many people decide to use chemicals in tablet form to increase their GH.

Until recently, it was not very clear whether these secretagogues acted directly on the pituitary and stimulated it to produce GH, or they acted indirectly on the hypothalamus to release GHRH which, in turn, stimulated GH production. In a recent experiment, scientists from Sao Paolo University in Brazil found that at least some of these secretagogues do indeed act directly on the pituitary receptors to stimulate GH release. This is important because it shows that the pituitary is still capable of producing GH and can respond to any signal sent either directly to it, or indirectly through GHRH. Taking secretagogues plus GHRH was shown to have maximum effects in some experimental animal studies. In addition, a few human trials show promising benefits from using this combination.

Pioneering experiments show that there are several sites within the brain tissues which are specifically aimed at binding secretagogues. Secretagogues home in on these sites, bind on to the cells and activate them. Receptors for secretagogues not only exist on the brain but also on other tissues, for example in the heart. Experiments with the secretagogue called hexarelin show that this molecule can have a direct beneficial effect on the heart, particularly when the treatment is prolonged, which has nothing to do with any GH released from the brain.

New brand-name secretagogues are being launched at an alarming rate. At the last count there were over 150 different products but the following are some of the more established.

> **Growth Hormone Releasing Peptide 6** (GHRP-6), a sequence of six amino acids, is the first synthetic secretagogue (hexarelin). It is one of the most well studied secretagogues but research results are conflicting. It was given to patients for a period of 16 weeks, in a study performed by researchers from the University of Manchester in the United Kingdom. The researchers concluded that hexarelin had no significant beneficial effects on muscle, fat content or bone strength. Taking hexarelin for a long period may also reduce those few benefits experienced originally, as the pituitary gets tired of the continuous stimulation and finally gives up. Whether this effect, called attenuation, is seen with other secretagogues is not clear but it is possible.

Other experiments show that GHRP-6 stimulates the release of GH in cycles which are similar to natural GH release cycles. Several experiments show some positive results from GHRP-6 use. In recent experiments, hexarelin-related compounds were shown to be effective in inducing penile erection in rats, if given by injection in the brain. This could be awkward if it proves to have the same effects in humans. Brain injections for impotence!

Symbiotropin (ProHGH) contains amino acid sequences, as well as plant-derived L-dopa and other plant chemicals which are said to regulate IGF1. It is thought to be effective in stimulating the pituitary through GHRH to secrete GH in pulses and thus mimics the natural pattern of GH release.

Meditropin is a stronger and more modern variant of the above, and is currently only available on a doctor's prescription. It contains symbiotropin and GHRH co-factors.

Ghrelin is a series of 28 amino acids formed in the stomach, so it is a natural variant. It is a strong GH releaser which works by binding to GH receptors and stimulating its effective release.

Somatomed, a secretagogue produced by Vespro Ltd., was found to be useful in chronic fatigue syndrome (CFS). Evaluation following the treatment of 200 patients suffering from CFS, showed that significant numbers of them experienced improvement in sleep patterns, better cognition, a decrease in muscle pain and fatigue. Side effects of this treatment were transient muscle pain and mild swelling of the hands and feet. **GHRH analogues or stimulants.** An experimental GHRH-analogue – i.e. a chemical having a similar structure to the original GHRH – has been found to be effective, and its actions persisted after long-term treatment. Among the advantages of the treatment were increasing IGF1 levels and many clinical improvements such as increased skin thickness, lean body mass and improved libido.

Other experimental secretagogues are so new that they have not even got proper names yet and are known only by their laboratory codes. For example, the one called NN703, is given by mouth and has similar effects to those of GHRP-6, as above. Another one called MK677 was found to have positive benefits on the bone, particularly helping to increase bone mass in the hip joint and to reduce the risk of osteoporosis.

Some secretagogues are enclosed in liposomes – minute special fat globules which can penetrate the skin and release any active substance they are carrying – for better absorption and can be given by oral spray. Individual substances which increase GH production, and many of these are included in the secretagogue combinations discussed above, are:

- the amino acid glutamine which increases GH secretion by 15%
- L-dopa, a drug used in Parkinson's disease, which is effective in men over 60 years old
- the amino acids arginine, lysine, and ornithine (usually at high doses of 2g daily)
- minerals such as potassium, zinc, magnesium, calcium, chromium and vanadium
- GABA, a type of amino acid
- homeopathic preparations of GH which are claimed to be able to stimulate GH release
- carnosine, possibly. It modulates the activity of the minerals zinc, magnesium, chromium and vanadium, which are thought to play a role in GH release. Also, although not yet proven, it is theoretically possible that carnosine is able to increase the sensitivity of the hypothalamus through special proteins and so protect and/or repair the receptors. If that is the case, carnosine would act as a 'hypothalamic and pituitary re-sensitizer', suitable for indirectly reactivating hormonal secretion by these two organs. There have been some animal experiments pointing us in the right direction. For example, it is known that carnosine modulates the

NMDA receptor in the brain, and regulates the actions of nitric oxide (NO) which, in turn, balances GH secretion. Incidentally, that is why the amino acid arginine is a good GH releaser, because it stimulates the production of NO.

OTHER RELEASERS OF GH

The Australian yeast extract Vegemite, similar to Marmite in the UK, was found to be a good GH releaser. These yeast extracts are effective in increasing GH production by about 30%, which is the average increase experienced from some of the synthetic secretagogues. There is anecdotal evidence that drinks such as Newcastle Brown Ale are potentially able to increase GH but the exact mechanism of this is still not clear. The drug GHB (gamma hydroxy butyrate) has been proven to have a strong releasing effect on GH, being able to cause an amazing 600% increase in GH secretion. GHB is, however, banned in several countries because it has the potential to be abused as a 'date rape' drug. Incidentally, GHB is believed by some doctors to be one of the best anti-ageing drugs available, if used properly.

SYNTHETIC GH VERSUS SECRETAGOGUES

GH is a promising anti-ageing treatment, but how to get it into the body is another matter. Artificial GH given by injection produces a 500–600% increase of GH in the body, but the treatment is expensive and has the potential for side effects. There is research showing that synthetic GH can be given not only by injection but also in nasal spray form or in patches, although more research is needed to support this.

Using secretagogues is also costly, and it may increase GH by only 30% but it is also less liable to cause side effects. People who choose to use secretagogues should make sure that the preparation they are using is at least partly supported by research. Some advertisements make it very confusing and difficult to get the real picture, claiming that a particular product is a real (synthetic or natural) GH molecule, when in fact it is only a poor quality secretagogue.

Certain claims made about secretagogues are completely invalid. Many products are advertised by gimmicky words such as 'revolutionary', 'unique', 'scientifically produced', 'ground-breaking'. The truth is that only some of these products have actually been found to be somewhat effective, and many of the rest are not well-studied substances.

Overall, some products may have measurable effects, whereas others may not. Scientific studies of these substances are few and far between, and the few studies that exist do not always show clear benefits. As things stand at the moment, it is a matter of getting as much information about the product as you can and deciding for yourself. If after, say, four to six months you do not experience any obvious benefits, then it may be time to stop using that particular product. As always, you should work together with your medical practitioner to find products which are suitable for you.

The bottom line is that injectable GH should only be used in selected cases under medical supervision. It is expensive and has the potential for side effects. Lower doses are better in the long term. Secretagogues are used by a wide section of the public but consideration should be given to the cost, the medical evidence supporting the particular secretagogue and the fact that there are no guarantees about the results. Remember that GH does not affect the underlying ageing process, but may improve some of the signs of ageing on the body.

CHAPTER 4

Co-enzyme Q10

Over and over again, nature comes up with chemical masterpieces which are deceptively simple but have an astonishing variety of benefits. Carnosine is one such compound, co-enzyme Q10 is another. These ingenious substances are 'pluripotent', in other words they are effective in many different biological processes and have multiple actions.

Co-enzyme Q10, or simply 'Q10', is one of the most abundant nutrients in your body. It is found in almost every tissue, and its description 'ubiquinone' attests to that. Its presence is 'ubiquitous' and, chemically, it belongs to the family of 'quinones'.

Your body soaks up some Q10 from food, but the average Q10 content of the Western diet is estimated at 100 times less than the amount your body actually needs for its everyday activities. Fortunately, your body is able to create new Q10 molecules under its own steam, to top up its supplies. However, this production of brand new Q10 becomes progressively less efficient with age, and here we encounter the old argument as to whether it is necessary to do something about this age-related deficiency, or just go along with nature's plan and leave things as they are. You will see that I support the former point of view and believe that, on balance, it is best to use extra Q10 supplements during ageing.

A MIGHTY ALLY

One of the main jobs of Q10 is to offer antioxidant protection. Q10 is present at the very heart of the metabolism, the mitochondria. It is able to quench any free radicals created by the mitochondria, which burn oxygen during the process of producing energy for fuelling the body. The mitochondria are the energy factories where the transformation of different chemicals produces energy. They utilize a tremendous amount of oxygen and so overproduction of free radicals is inevitable. Trouble is always brewing inside the mitochondria. The presence of Q10 within the mitochondria is nature's way of dealing with these excessive free radicals, which need to be inactivated before they can cause any serious mischief.

Excessive free radical production speeds up the process of apoptosis which results in the death of too many normal cells. As I have explained before, a moderate degree of apoptosis is necessary to get rid of any damaged cells with minimal disruption to the surrounding cells, but an accelerated apoptosis eliminates so many cells that those left behind become unable to cope with their normal duties. This leaves the tissues in shambles. Q10, being 50 times stronger than vitamin E, protects against this extreme cell death by reducing the cell exposure to free radicals.

Your mitochondria come furnished with their own special DNA supply which needs to be protected as efficiently as the rest of your DNA. Normally, the DNA molecule in the central nucleus of the cells is relatively well protected against the rigours of ageing, but the DNA which is inside the mitochondria is exposed to an immense amount of free radical hits and it is liable to be easily damaged. In fact, many scientists believe that injury to the mitochondrial DNA is one of the first signs seen during the ageing process. Drastic measures are needed here, and Q10 comes to the rescue.

Several experiments done on mice show that Q10 is able to protect mitochondrial DNA from this kind of damage. The very latest studies report that Q10 supplements may also protect human mitochondrial DNA from free radical attack. This is good news, because damaged DNA can build up over time. This disrupts the normal workings of the mitochondria, causing a 'power meltdown', eventually resulting in ageing and early death.

CO-ENZYME Q10 AS AN ENERGISER

In addition to its antioxidant activity, Q10 is also very accomplished at boosting overall energy and muscle strength. It facilitates the production of chemical energy from the burning of oxygen inside the mitochondria. Scientists who studied the effects of Q10 on rats, found that it can protect the animals' capacity to respond to stress and improves their muscle endurance.

When experimenting with heart tissue from people with heart disease, scientists discovered that young cells normally recover much faster than older cells following stress, such as the lack of oxygen. However, when these cells were pretreated with Q10, the difference between young and old was abolished, and the older cells recovered as quickly as the young ones. Amazing isn't it! This shows that Q10 may have a role to play in maintaining the muscle metabolism in older people when the blood supply is interrupted, during a heart attack, for example.

Q10 AND HEART DISEASE

The concentration of Q10 in the heart muscle plummets with age, and is usually lower in patients who have heart disease than in those of similar age without any heart problems. Several properly performed scientific trials have shown that Q10 is effective in reducing some of the symptoms of stroke, heart failure, heart attack and angina.

It works like this. The 'bad' fat, LDL (low density lipoprotein), carries cholesterol around the body via the bloodstream. Free radical damage to LDL is an important cause of atherosclerosis, which is thickening of the arteries and may result in heart problems and stroke. Vitamin E and Q10 are the antioxidants which play a serious part in reducing the union between free radicals and LDL within the blood vessels and so reduce the risk of atherosclerosis. Studies performed both in animals and in humans have proved that Q10 is particularly useful in this situation and that it can be used to prevent heart disease in the long term.

Other experiments show that taking 150 mg of Q10 a day is effective at slashing the frequency of angina pain almost by half. Also, if Q10 is given to patients who undergo a heart operation, it considerably reduces the amount of injury to the heart muscle, both during and after the operation.

Vitamin E – Friend or Foe?

The use of vitamin E on its own may, for some strange reason, worsen free radical attack on LDL on certain occasions. This process is called 'tocopherol-mediated peroxidation'—remember that vitamin E is also called tocopherol. In this case, vitamin E behaves not as an anti-oxidant, but as a pro-oxidant. The presence of Q10 though, protects against this worrying phenomenon and turns vitamin E back to behave as an anti-oxidant again.

So, vitamin E and Q10 need to be taken together, ideally in a single combination tablet, for maximum protection against lipid peroxidation. Experiments confirm that Q10 plus vitamin E is a more effective strategy against atherosclerosis than Q10 or vitamin E given separately.

As I mentioned earlier, the chemical nitric oxide (NO) if left unbalanced may play a significant role during inflammation which may well contribute to atherosclerosis. A toxic byproduct of nitric oxide called 'peroxynitrite', can be kept at bay by using Q10 supplements. Patients who were treated with a daily dose of 150 mg of Q10 for five days, had a decreased amount of peroxynitrite in their blood which means that their risk of developing atherosclerosis and, consequently, heart problems, was reduced.

This was confirmed by another experiment using animal brain tissue, which showed that both NO and our old friend MDA (malondialdehyde) are kept low after toxic injury, but only if the brain is treated with very large doses of Q10. The benefits shown in animal experiments have also been confirmed during human clinical trials. Several studies using relatively high doses of Q10 (150 mg–600 mg) showed that heart disease patients may experience an improvement in their angina, with an ability to walk further than usual and a reduced need for medication.

In some of these trials, the blood levels of other anti-oxidants (such as vitamin E and vitamin C) were increased as if by magic, even though Q10 was the only nutrient supplied. This means that Q10 may have the ability to fuel the production of other antioxidants in the body.

Apart from its use in reducing the symptoms of angina, Q10 is also useful in rectifying heart failure, and several experiments support this. Heart failure patients may experience many symptoms including:

- shortness of breath
- swelling of the legs
- tiredness
- blue or pale extremities
- loss of appetite

I am not, of course, suggesting that Q10 can make these symptoms disappear completely but it may improve the overall condition, particularly when taken in association with conventional drugs.

Patients who use cholesterol-lowering drugs called statins, may benefit from Q10 supplements, because it is believed that some of these statin drugs block the actions of Q10. When Q10 is given as an additional supplement, however, the statins and Q10 work together to lower cholesterol even further. Having said that, trials with the cholesterol-lowering drugs called 'pravastatin' and 'atorvastatin' have shown that these two do not always decrease Q10, so people who take these two particular drugs may not need to take additional Q10 supplements. Atorvastatin has, in fact, been withdrawn in some countries due to fears that it may cause muscle problems.

New studies also show that Q10 reduces abnormally high blood pressure. In a typical study, 59 patients with high blood pressure were given either 120 mg of Q10 or a placebo for two months. The Q10 group experienced a fall in blood pressure, and a decrease of LDL, together with an increase in the 'good' fat HDL. Q10 was also able to reduce blood glucose and improve the ability of insulin to deal with glucose more effectively. This is good news because, as I have already explained, too much glucose in the blood contributes to glycation and AGE formation.

Case Study

The benefits of Q10 in limiting brain damage after the oxygen supply is cut off are well known. This makes it a promising supplement to use in stroke. In a discussion about the anti-stroke benefits of Q10, I was told of a woman who was taking 400 mg of Q10 a day when she had a head injury resulting in a stroke. She was in coma and was expected to die within a few days, but she recovered after ten days. Was this because her brain was protected by the Q10? Maybe. Other similar unsubstantiated cases have also been reported.

MACULAR DEGENERATION

This age-related condition is one of the most common causes of partial blindness in the world. It is thought to be, at least in part, due to free radicals attacking the retina at the back of the eye.

In a recent study, Italian scientists measured the Q10 content of the blood in patients with macular degeneration and found it to be lower than that of healthy people of the same age. Patients with macular degeneration were also less able to deal with free radicals than healthy people. The researchers concluded that Q10 supplements may well protect against macular degeneration.

CANCER

Unconfirmed experiments show that Q10 may be effective in reducing the advance of cancers, such as those of the prostate and breast. The concentration of Q10 in the blood of people suffering from prostate or breast cancer is low anyway, but giving high doses of Q10 to such patients reduces some of the effects of these cancers. For example, it lowers the level of PSA in prostate cancer, high PSA or prostatic specific antigen being a general sign that cancer of the prostate is a possibility. But these are small trials and larger ones are needed. If this anti-cancer potential of Q10 proves to be case, then Q10 will be an ideal partner to use with DHEA which may, in some instances, worsen the risk of prostate or breast cancer.

Although Q10 was found to protect the heart during certain types of chemotherapy for cancer, particularly if used in association with vitamin E, its widespread use during chemotherapy is not generally recommended, in case it worsens free radical activity during the treatment. Again, more research is needed to clarify this.

BRAIN HEALTH

Q10 treatment helps improve brain function. This is achieved in a variety of ways:

- It protects against free radicals which are massing to unleash their power onto the brain cells. If left uncontrolled, this destruction could result in the production of beta amyloid which is found in the brain of Alzheimer's disease patients.
- It limits overproduction of glutamate which may cause excitotoxicity, the brain injury caused by too much stimulation.
- Q10 improves the general metabolism of brain cells.

Some patients with Parkinson's disease have a low Q10 concentration in their brains. This, some scientists speculate, suggests that Q10 supplements may help lessen some of the symptoms of the disease.

GUM HEALTH

Q10 is used by some people in oral spray form to prevent and treat gum disease. It reduces gum bleeding and helps maintain healthy gum tissues. Gum disease is one of the commonest problems related to ageing, and it is this that causes the loss of teeth. Japanese researchers found that Q10 reduces swelling and pain of the gums. Some people apply the oil from Q10 capsules directly on to their gums, but the spray for direct application on the gums, or the tablets taken by mouth are also effective.

GENERAL ENERGY AND MUSCULAR CONDITIONS

Many of my patients who take Q10 supplements experience an increase in their levels of energy. This makes them more active and reduces feelings of tiredness. Q10 is also used to fight several conditions which cause muscle weakness such as muscular dystrophy, multiple sclerosis, and other myopathies because it improves energy in the muscle and protects the mitochondria. However, sufferers from these conditions are generally advised by their practitioner to take Q10 in higher doses than usual.

You will remember that growth hormone or DHEA are also used by some sufferers of muscular conditions. Combining Q10 with growth hormone or with DHEA may bestow stronger benefits on some of these patients.

A Skin Rejuvenator

The health-supporting properties of Q10 make it a convenient substance for the cosmetic industry to use. Creams containing Q10 are marketed as being effective in reducing the results of skin ageing. Q10 is used with other products for maximum anti-ageing support to the skin. Examples of these are:

aloe vera

antioxidants

retinol

DHEA/melatonin complexes

HOW TO TAKE CO-ENZYME Q10

Q10 needs to be taken with some form of fat, because its absorption is enhanced in the presence of fat in the diet. There are capsules containing Q10 mixed with oil and these are thought to be more suitable than simple tablets. It is important to choose good quality Q10 which means that it has to be of the expensive pharmaceutical grade quality, and standardized to provide equal amounts of Q10 with every capsule.

I have already mentioned that it is best to take it together with vitamin E, and many preparations do indeed contain this vitamin within the same capsule as the Q10. The available preparations come in different strengths, commonly 10 mg, 30 mg and 100 mg. Most people who take 30 mg of Q10 are adequately covered but there are others who take higher doses without any side effects.

IDEBENONE

This is a close variant of Q10, which is claimed to possess a wider range of benefits than Q10 itself. It is stronger than Q10 and affords a better protection against free radicals. It is a generally more efficient chemical than Q10.

Its antioxidant actions have aroused interest in the treatment of brain problems such as dementia. In a German trial, a six month course of 90 mg of idebenone a day was found to create a significant improvement in patients with Alzheimer's disease. It improved memory, attention span, and orientation and it slowed down the natural progression of Alzheimer's, albeit temporarily. This is because it offers protection to the membrane of the nerve cells, enhances the speed of information transmission, and powers up the brain metabolism. It encourages the production of nerve growth factors which are needed for the normal grooming of the nerve cells.

Some people recommend taking both Q10 and idebenone for maximum benefits. Side effects are mild nausea, anxiety and sleep difficulties. Remember that both Q10 and idebenone are energy-boosters and increase general metabolism. The normal dose is 45 mg once or twice a day, but double this amount can be used for specific diseases. Idebenone can be taken with a wide variety of other anti-ageing drugs for best effects.

The bottom line is that Q10 is cheap and easily available. Its actions are multiple and a good deal of the research is positive. It is becoming increasingly accepted by medical practitioners in general. Do remember that it is best taken together with vitamin E and other antioxidants.

CHAPTER 5

Methylation Enhancers

Without methylation you will die in a matter of days. Defective methylation is a time bomb, and the biological clock of those who cannot repair this deficiency is about to run down.

Faulty methylation causes several problems, but one of the most important is the increase of homocysteine which worsens the risk of developing a number of age-related diseases. Homocysteine is a type of amino acid, a by-product of another amino acid, methionine. Whereas methionine is essential to your health, as it takes part in many normal processes, homocysteine is exactly the opposite, having been associated with illness, as we shall see below.

THE STREAKER'S CYCLE

Homocysteine is methionine without its clothes on, a kind of streaker causing disruption during the game of life. It is what remains when good methionine is used by the tissues to methylate your proteins and DNA. Normally, as soon as homocysteine is formed, it is quickly clothed with methyl groups and converted back to methionine again.

Folic acid, vitamins of the B group and the chemical SAMe (see below) are needed for this conversion to take place. They are the police officers and the clothes-bearers who cover homocysteine up quickly, before disorder can become unmanageable. Homocysteine can also be transformed through several steps into a very useful antioxidant, glutathione, again with the help of vitamins of the B group. This cycle continues over and over again throughout life.

If, for any reason, any of the steps of this cycle are disturbed, then homocysteine cannot adequately revert to useful methionine or even to glutathione, and so it remains behind ready to cause trouble. I do not know if you have ever been into a stadium with several streakers running loose for hours. I have not, but I can imagine what happens. Everything must end in total chaos.

One reason for the defective operation of the methionine-homocysteine cycle is lack of folic acid and a deficiency of vitamins of the B group, such as vitamin B6 and B12. When these vitamins are low in your tissues, the homocysteine cycle misfires and becomes unable to operate at full speed. Too much homocysteine is created but it cannot be quickly covered up and inactivated.

The problem is that these vitamins become progressively less effective with age, even in healthy older people. It is as if these molecular policemen become too sluggish to run after the streakers. In addition, any deficiency of these vitamins in your diet will make matters worse, the equivalent of not supplying enough police officers or clothes during the game. Consuming folic acid and B vitamins is essential in keeping the cycle of homocysteine going. These vitamins should be obtained mainly from green vegetables and fruit. The mineral zinc is also used somewhere in this process, to make matters a bit easier. It is a kind of a policeman's hat which covers the sensitive parts of the streaker until further help arrives. Zinc is obtained from oysters, pulses, wholegrain cereals and lean beef which, as we have seen, is also a good source of carnosine.

Why, you may ask, is it necessary for 'nice' methionine to be transformed to noxious homocysteine in the first place? The answer is that methionine is needed to methylate other essential molecules down the line, such as proteins, enzymes, DNA, phospholipids and so on. During this process, methionine creates methyl groups which are picked up by carrier chemicals such as SAMe, and then taken to those constituents of your body which consume methyl groups for their own maintenance.

Homocysteine is a necessary by-product of this process, and it is meant to be inactivated quickly thereafter. But, as we have seen, things do not always work as smoothly, and homocysteine can stay behind. High levels of homocysteine mean that the methylation processes in the body are below par. The body is able to deal with defective methylation for a short while, but not for long.

HEART DISEASE

Health conditions which are thought to be aggravated by high homocysteine include heart disease and stroke. There are several reasons for this:

- homocysteine encourages the clumping together of platelets resulting in abnormal clotting of blood.
- It makes it more difficult for the arteries to relax as it interferes with nitric oxide which normally keeps the blood vessels nice and wide, and therefore causes obstruction of the normal blood flow.
- In the mitochondria of the heart muscle cells, homocysteine interacts with iron and copper metal ions to speed up production of free radicals. These, in turn, encourage 'bad' fat LDL to cause even more oxidation-related damage.

Eventually, heart attack, stroke and other circulation problems, such as thrombosis of the legs and lungs, become more likely. Problems related to high homocysteine are particularly likely to happen in people aged 50 and over, perhaps due to the fact that the nutrients which limit homocysteine, such as vitamin B, become less abundant with age. High homocysteine is considered by doctors to be a risk factor for heart disease, equally as important as other heart disease risk factors such as smoking, lack of exercise and obesity.

DEMENTIA

There are concerns that high homocysteine in the blood plays a part in causing Alzheimer's disease. Alzheimer's disease patients have low levels of folic acid in their brain, which may be a sign that the homocysteine cycle is blocked. A Swedish study of 370 people aged over 75 years, found that those with low levels of folic acid and vitamin B12 were at an increased risk of developing Alzheimer's. At the same time, those who had high levels of these two vitamins were at a low risk.

The chemical SAMe which helps reduce the amounts of homocysteine, is usually low in the brain of Alzheimer's disease patients. Homocysteine can also damage the lining of the nerves and this is seen particularly in patients who have diabetes.

LIVER DISEASE

Researchers trying to clarify the actions of homocysteine have shown that this chemical can cause liver problems. This could be due to the pro-oxidant activity of homocysteine as it helps create free radicals which attack the liver cells.

Homocysteine also interferes with the liver enzymes. Alcohol causes liver damage and, apart from the toxic effects of alcohol directly on to the liver cells, this damage is also explained by the fact that alcohol reduces the amounts of B vitamins in the liver.

DEPRESSION

High homocysteine has been associated with depression. This is because the chemical serotonin, which reduces the symptoms of depression, needs to be constantly methylated in order to keep up its good work. Slow methylation results in inactive serotonin which cannot work properly in the brain, resulting in depression. A sign of low methylation is high homocysteine.

You will see below that chemicals such as SAMe which encourage methylation may improve serotonin levels which, in turn, decrease depression, as well as reduce homocysteine. You can see here how one chemical affects another, just like hormones which affect one another. Deficiency of one chemical causes repercussions right through the entire system.

AGEING

The ageing process itself may be affected by homocysteine. The telomeres (the end parts of the DNA molecule) are usually damaged by free radicals and start shrinking with age. Short telomeres are one of the signs of ageing. It was found that homocysteine accelerates this process of telomere destruction. The exact explanation why this happens is not very clear at present, but it implies that nutrients which reduce homocysteine may well have a protective effect on telomeres.

HOW TO DEAL WITH HOMOCYSTEINE

So far I have mentioned some of the problems encountered when there are high homocysteine levels. But what can you do about all of this? Is there a way to help yourself?

It is possible to have blood tests for homocysteine and to assess whether you are at risk. The higher the value of homocysteine, the higher the risk of disease. The good news is that homocysteine can be reduced, and that methylation can be increased by simple changes in your diet and by taking the right supplements. The best diet to reduce homocysteine is a combination diet containing:

- low fat dairy products
- fruits and vegetables
- fish
- dry cereals
- small quantities of lean pork and beef.

Factors and chemicals which adjust and modulate methylation are used by many millions of people across the world. Two main examples of these, apart from vitamins of the B group, are SAMe and TMG.

SAME

In my book *Stay Young Longer – Naturally* (Vega Publishers, 2001) I considered SAMe to be one of the essential ingredients of the 'elixir of youth'. I still do. SAMe stands for S-Adenosyl-Methionine and it is a natural chemical found in all living cells. It is a result of the union between the amino acid methionine and the energy chemical ATP (adenosine triphosphate). SAMe plays a serious part in promoting healthy methylation, as well as helping the body to produce sufficient quantities of the antioxidant glutathione and hence reduce the overall concentration of homocysteine.

Any reduction of the vitamins B6, B12 and of folic acid disrupts the normal metabolism of SAMe and therefore may increase homocysteine and reduce useful glutathione. Conditions that may reduce the normal amounts of SAMe in the body include:

- dementia
- liver disease
- depression
- alcoholism
- the ageing process in general.

It is not exactly known whether these conditions are the cause or the result of low SAMe, but research will clarify this point in the next few years. Whatever the situation, these conditions are irrevocably associated with high homocysteine and anything that lowers homocysteine also improves SAMe. Most of the actions of SAMe are the exact opposites of the actions of homocysteine.

SAME AND DEPRESSION

Many doctors practising alternative medicine say that SAMe is one of the most effective and safe antidepressants available. Clinical trials have found that SAMe is as effective in relieving depression as the prescription-only antidepressant imipramine, and it does not have its side effects. The antidepressant actions of SAMe have also been studied in comparison with other prescription antidepressants and found to be equal or superior in many cases.

SAMe versus Herbs

SAMe is sometimes compared to herbal antidepressants or brain nutrients such as:

St John's wort

kava kava

ginseng

ginkgo biloba

However, SAMe is even more natural than herbal antidepressants.

Herbal chemicals are obviously not as natural for humans as they are for plants. It is more natural for people to use something like SAMe which is found in all human cells, in preference to something that is found only in plants.

SAMe is also suitable for treating depression resulting from illnesses such as alcoholism, fibromyalgia and chronic arthritis. It is useful not only in curing the actual condition but also in relieving the depression which is caused as a result of that condition. SAMe helps increase the brain chemical serotonin which as I have mentioned is responsible for improving the symptoms of depression.

Serotonin helps to keep you awake and active, and it is more efficient during the day. It could be considered the opposite of melatonin which is useful for inducing sleep and which works during the night. SAMe is needed to adjust this balance between serotonin and melatonin and therefore it helps maintain a healthy sleeping – waking cycle.

The way SAMe works is by helping serotonin bind easily to the cell receptors. It also improves the function of the cell membrane by increasing production of phosphatidyl choline, one of its essential constituents. SAMe is one of the most important methylating agents in the brain. Loss of brain methylation has not only been blamed for depression but is also associated with ageing in general.

THE LIVER

SAMe helps protect the liver against alcohol and other toxic damage. Drugs which destroy the liver cells include oestrogens, anti-inflammatories and painkillers, but SAMe shields the liver against these. Supplements which support the actions of SAMe in the liver are silymarin, vitamin E and lipoic acid.

ARTHRITIS

Some patients suffering from joint problems and arthritis have been using SAMe with good results. In experiments it was found to improve the structure of the cartilage and thus relieve some of the problems related to osteoarthritis.

As long ago as 1987 over 22,000 patients took part in clinical trials evaluating the benefits of SAMe in arthritis, so it is a relatively well studied remedy. It is used by people who have other forms of arthritis such as rheumatoid arthritis, as well as by those with fibromyalgia, osteoporosis and joint injuries. As opposed to certain anti-inflammatories, SAMe is able to protect the lining of the stomach against acid injury, whereas some anti-inflammatories may actually damage the lining of the stomach. It can be used in association with the anti-arthritis nutrients chondroitin and glucosamine for joint support.

DOSE

Dosage depends on the problems being treated.

- Higher doses are usually needed in depression – 200 mg–400 mg twice a day initially and then increasing to three or four times a day.
- Similar or even higher strengths are used for patients with liver problems and arthritis. People usually start with a low dose and increase it as necessary.
- For general anti-ageing and methylation support the average dose is 200 mg–400 mg once or twice daily.

SAMe is quite expensive in the long term but costs are expected to fall when better ways of manufacturing it are found. Taking extra supplements of a cheaper chemical called TMG (see below) may reduce the necessity for taking the full dose of SAMe which brings the cost down appreciably. TMG and SAMe work together, complementing each other. The 'enteric coated' tablets are manufactured specifically for better absorption and they should not be cut in half, nor should they be exposed to sunlight.

Side effects are rare, but include occasional nausea and stomach upset. The side effects are generally well tolerated and improve after a while. In one experiment SAMe was proven to be free from significant side effects after two years of continuous use.

In another experiment involving 734 participants, only 10 people had mild side effects due to SAMe whereas 13 people apparently had side effects just by taking the dummy treatment, or placebo. People who suffer from the manic form of depression should not use SAMe because it makes the condition worse.

TMG

Tri-Methyl-Glycine (TMG, also called 'betaine') is another methylating agent. As the name suggests, TMG has three methyl groups which are easily donated to other structures in need of methylation, particularly the DNA. Donating a methyl group to homocysteine transforms it into the useful amino acid methionine as explained above. In theory, because it can help lower homocysteine, it also reduces the risk of heart attacks and stroke.

Side effects include mild headaches or muscle tension at high doses, but these usually improve after reducing the dose. It comes in 500 mg tablets and in powder form and it should be taken in association with vitamins B6 and B12 to help maintain the methylating cycle of homocysteine.

A Summary of Methylation

Although the workings of the methylation cycle appear convoluted, in reality they are not. Several illnesses which are related to methylation become more likely when methylation is slow, and may improve when methylation is speeded up. Nutrients such as SAMe, TMG and vitamin B keep this process going and so reduce the likelihood of methylation-dependant diseases.

A sign of how active the methylation processes are in the body is given by homocysteine. If homocysteine is high, it means that methylation is defective. If it is normal, it means that methylation is fine.

SAMe, vitamins of the B group and other methylating nutrients need to be taken both in the diet and in supplements. SAMe can be expensive however. These nutrients help prevent or treat certain age-related illness, but do not, as a rule, appear to reverse the underlying rate of ageing.

CHAPTER 6

Adaptogens

A large percentage of all chronic degenerative diseases of ageing is believed to occur because people suffer high levels of stress which last for long periods at a time. Modern living is synonymous with high stress and this is probably the main factor causing chronic disease and premature ageing. Fortunately, Mother Nature has an answer to this challenge – a unique class of herbal products called 'adaptogens'. These herbal remedies have a wide range of healing properties, but their unique value is that they specifically relieve stress.

Before discussing some of these adaptogens, I want to highlight certain facts about stress.

The three phases of stress are:

> ***Alarm phase –*** When your body experiences a stressful event, there is a sudden release of powerful stress-hormones such as steroids and catecholamines. If the stress is very intense it can damage the way these hormones are being produced and it can interfere with how they affect your body.

Adaptation phase – If the stress continues as with heavy athletic training, or intense pressure to meet deadlines at work, for example, your body learns to tolerate the stressful stimulation, and it adapts and increases its resistance to the stress factor. The 'adaptation phase' is usually a safe period. The longer you can stay in the 'adaptation phase', the better.

Exhaustion phase – This finally appears when your body fails to fight stress any more and simply gives up. In this 'exhaustion phase' disease symptoms appear quite quickly and may worsen in the long term.

Although some illnesses associated with stress may appear in the first 'alarm phase', the majority appear in the third 'exhaustion phase' when the organism cannot fight stress any longer. This 'exhaustion phase' usually develops after a period of months or years of stress. Everything depends on the duration of the 'adaptation phase'. On occasions, you may be lucky and escape the third phase altogether, provided that you can keep the stress under control. Certain health practitioners suggest that you may be able to achieve this by taking adaptogens which can help you stay in the 'adaptation phase' for as long as possible.

The main benefits of adaptogens are that they increase energy during everyday metabolism, and maintain the body in the 'adaptation phase' of stress. Other benefits are:

- a reduction in the levels of stress
- increased endurance and muscle power
- better mental function
- deep and relaxing sleep

Adaptogens also significantly accelerate the recovery process after an illness. According to modern science, adaptogens are natural plant products that increase the body's ability to cope with internal and external stress factors, and balance the everyday functioning of your body. They help maintain the stable environment – known as homeostasis – inside the organism. An important characteristic is that they are safe, possessing few known side effects. Nevertheless, they should be taken only under medical or expert supervision.

You are probably already familiar with the names of some common adaptogens such as Panax ginseng, American ginseng, and Siberian ginseng, but in this chapter I will also discuss certain less well known ones. All of them may be helpful in improving your chances of achieving healthy and stress-less ageing.

GINSENG

Korean and Chinese ginseng (Panax), Siberian ginseng (eleutherococcus) and American ginseng (Panax quinquefolius) are used widely for anti-ageing purposes in general, and also against atherosclerosis, diabetes, depression, loss of energy, and sleep problems. The active ingredients help improve the actions of the neurotransmitter acetylcholine, which is involved in memory function. They also protect the brain against free radical damage and neutralize toxic material in the brain. American ginseng was shown to reduce the 'bad' cholesterol LDL and it also increases the release of nitric oxide (NO) and thus plays an important part in protecting against circulation problems. It has mild oestrogen effects on the body so it may increase vaginal bleeding, though Siberian ginseng may cause less interference with menstruation. Those with high blood pressure and an irregular heart beat should avoid ginseng.

RHODIOLA ROSEA (RUSSIAN RHODIOLA)

Rhodiola is a powerful anti-ageing plant supplement with proven anti-stress effectiveness. In Russia, Rhodiola rosea, also known as 'golden root', has been used for centuries to help people cope with the cold Siberian climate and stressful life. It is a perennial plant with red, pink, or yellowish flowers. One of the greatest benefits of Rhodiola is its ability to enhance mental and physical performance. It has been widely used by Russian athletes and cosmonauts to increase energy during physically and mentally demanding tasks. Rhodiola is cardio-protective, normalizing the heart rate immediately after intense exercise. It also improves the nervous system and mental functions such as memory by increasing the supply of blood to your muscles and your brain.

The antidepressant and anti-stress activity of Rhodiola is greater than that of St. John's wort, Ginkgo biloba and Panax ginseng. Also, it has been calculated that Rhodiola rosea is five times less likely to cause side effects than Panax ginseng. In a clinical trial, 150 individuals suffering from depression took Rhodiola extracts for a period of one month. At the end of that period two thirds of the patients reported a full remission of clinical signs of depression, and that they had become more active and more sociable. General weakness also disappeared.

There are many products on the market that contain Rhodiola rosea. Unfortunately, these products often have limited or even no biological activity. Common reasons for these deficiencies are the use of the incorrect species of plant, cultivating it in the wrong geographic area or at the wrong time of the year, harvesting at the wrong season, over-drying, or using an inferior extraction method. The main active components of true Rhodiola rosea that are responsible for its potency are cinnamol alcohol glycosides (rosavin and salidroside). Quality Rhodiola rosea extract should contain at least 2% rosavin and 1% salidroside.

Rhodiola rosea of Russian origin is now slowly becoming more widely accepted in Europe and the United States as a powerful anti-ageing, anti-stress formula for the 21st century. It is in our interest to take advantage of this powerful herb if we want to survive the demands modern life imposes on us.

Dose: You can prepare this for personal use in the following way: mill 30 gm of Rhodiola rosea roots in a coffee grinder, add 150 ml of vodka without aromatic additives, agitate and keep for 3-5 days at room temperature. Separate and filter the extract. Take half a teaspoonful 3 times a day.

ASHWAGANDHA

A herb used in ancient Indian Ayurvedic medicine, ashwagandha is also known as Withania somnifera. It is thought to have anti-stress properties, increasing muscle strength and physical resistance. People have used it as:

- an aphrodisiac
- an anti-inflammatory
- an anti-arthritis medication
- a memory boosting medication.

It contains several active plant chemicals such as alkaloids, withanolides and sitoindosides. It is sometimes used in association with other herbal extracts which work together to increase each others' benefits. Ashwagandha is employed in the area of Ayurvedic medicine which offers rasayana or rejuvenation therapies, aiming to treat body and mind. Any part of the plant can be used, although it is the root which is used most frequently.

Indian scientists from the Department of Zoology at Kurukshetra University have found that ashwagandha boosts antioxidants and reduces free radical damage to the fatty parts of the cells (lipid peroxidation). In addition, it protects proteins against toxic damage, leading the scientists to conclude that 'the plant has a therapeutic potential in ageing...'

Other Indian researchers studied the effects of ashwagandha on the brain of laboratory animals. They found that the plant improves memory and learning. Its benefits are thought to be due to its ability to enhance the concentration of acetylcholine, which is a neurotransmitter – a substance which helps to transmit information from one part of the brain to another.

Ashwagandha is also used against anxiety, to improve mood and behaviour. In an experiment, the effectiveness of extracts of the root of the plant was compared to that of the well-known anti-anxiety medication, lorazepam, and to the antidepressant imipramine. The results showed that ashwagandha was at least as effective as these two prescription-only drugs, confirming that it can be used as a mood stabilizer in anxiety and depression.

Finally, a review of the known actions of ashwagandha concluded that the plant has a wide variety of therapeutic benefits with no associated toxicity or side effects. The authors concluded: 'These results are very encouraging and indicate that this herb should be studied more extensively to reveal other potential benefits.'

Dose: The dose is 330 mg in capsule form, taken 3 times a day. The root can also be used in dry powder form, with 1 gm-10 gm dissolved in boiling water and drunk twice a day.

TARAXACUM

Another example of an effective adaptogen is Taraxacum officinale, more commonly known as dandelion extract. This has been studied extensively during the past few years and many positive reports about its activities have been published in scientific journals. Taraxacum officinale, dandelion, is a perennial weed found in many countries across the world. For some reason, it is also known as 'swine's snout'. It has shiny dark green leaves with golden yellow flowers.

In traditional medicine, the roots of the taraxacum plant are used against jaundice and for gall bladder problems, whereas the leaves are used specifically to reduce fluid retention. Taraxacum contains several plant chemicals, such as terpenoids and sterols which are also found in many other plants. But there are certain plant chemicals which are found only in taraxacum. Examples of these are the substances called taraxacin, taraxacerin and taraxinic acid. These plant chemicals have several beneficial actions, the most important of which is a possible effect on cancer of the blood, leukaemia.

Korean scientists from the College of Pharmacy at Kyung Heen University in Seoul have reported that taraxinic acid is especially active against cancerous cells obtained from patients with leukaemia. Dr Choi, the principal investigator, concluded that: 'taraxinic acid may have a potential as a therapeutic agent in human leukaemia.'

In addition to the above, taraxacum extract also contains other beneficial chemicals such as:

- flavonoids
- vitamins A, C and D
- resin and mucilage
- minerals such as magnesium, iron, potassium
- inulin and other polysaccharides.

These work together to produce taraxacum's multiple health benefits. One such benefit is its antioxidant activity. Canadian researchers from the Faculty of Agricultural Sciences at the University of British Columbia have studied the antioxidant effects of an extract from taraxacum flowers. They reported that the extract produces typical antioxidant benefits.

Specifically, it protects against DNA damage caused by free radicals, and reduces free-radical damage to the fat components of your cells, particularly if used at high doses. This highlights the need for further scientific studies with human volunteers to confirm this potentially ground-breaking, anti-ageing and anti-cancer benefit of taraxacum.

The inulin content of taraxacum helps prevent excessive glucose levels in the blood. Inulin – not to be confused with insulin, which is a hormone – is a type of fibre which traps glucose molecules and does not allow them to go over a certain safe limit in the blood. So it is a useful remedy against diabetes. Dr R Petlevski and his team at the Department of Medical Biochemistry and Haematology at the University of Zagreb in Croatia, have studied the effects of taraxacum and other plant extracts on diabetic mice. They found that preparations containing taraxacum extracts are effective at reducing excessively high glucose levels in the blood by up to 20 %. This reduction was apparent just two hours after administration of taraxacum, which shows that this plant can work almost immediately. In addition, Dr Petlevski found that taraxacum continued to be effective at reducing blood sugar when the treatment was given for a whole week.

Most diuretics (water retention remedies) cause a loss of the mineral potassium from the kidneys. This may well result in abnormalities of the heart rhythm and in muscle weakness. The good news is that taraxacum actually preserves potassium when it is used as a diuretic, helping the body to eliminate unwanted fluids. This is useful for people who are trying to lose weight, those with high blood pressure or those who suffer from excessive fluid retention which can cause swollen ankles, difficulty in breathing and a swollen stomach.

New research is revealing several hitherto unknown benefits of taraxacum. For example, Korean researchers from the Department of Biological Sciences at the University of Ulsan have reported their discovery of a protein molecule present in taraxacum, which acts as an anticoagulant. This protein stops the blood from clotting prematurely and could therefore be used in preventing blood clots which cause strokes, heart attacks and thrombosis of the leg veins. Another benefit of taraxacum is that it blocks chemicals which cause inflammation. Specifically, interleukin-6 and tumour necrosis factor-alpha (TNF-a) are implicated in causing inflammation reactions which result in cancer, arthritis and brain damage. However, taraxacum extracts have the ability to block both interleukin-6 and TNF-a, thus reducing the likelihood of chronic disease.

Dose: The dose is 500 mg 2 to 8 times daily. There are no reports of side effects or toxicity, but in very rare instances people who are allergic to pollen may also be allergic to taraxacum extract.

SCHISANDRA CHINENSIS

In the wild meadows of north China grows a woody, thorny vine with small berries. The berries, being very bright red, are so noticeable that they have attracted the attention of healers and physicians for almost six thousand years. This thorny plant is known locally as Wu Wei Tzu and in the West as Schisandra chinensis (Chinese magnolia). The ancient Chinese – as recorded in medical texts dated 2697 BC – believed Schisandra to be very effective in improving energy levels, boosting muscle power, stimulating memory, improving resistance against infections, and reducing stress.

Today, Schisandra is classified as an adaptogen. Modern science shows that adaptogens have exactly the same properties as those discovered by the ancient Chinese. Adaptogens are now being evaluated with regards to their action in protecting the liver, reducing anxiety and stress, stimulating the immune system which fights infections, improving mental well-being and enhancing physical performance. So much so, that Russian Olympic athletes have frequently, and legally, used Schisandra, to optimize their performance.

Over the past two or three years there has been tremendous scientific interest in adaptogens, and several dozen technical reports have been published on Schisandra chinensis alone. These positive reports come from all over the world, including China and the United States.

Biochemical technicians working at the College of Chemistry and Chemical Engineering of the Hunan University in China, have found that Schisandra chinensis contains several hitherto unknown chemical ingredients which have a variety of health boosting benefits. They discovered a special technical method to identify and extract these ingredients, making it easier for other scientists to examine the benefits of Schisandra in more detail.

Examples of Schisandra's active ingredients include:

- schisandrin A, B and C
- schisandrol
- gomisin

All of these are lignans, powerful plant chemicals that regulate the metabolism, balance the hormones and protect the constituents of your cells against injury or toxins.

Scientists working at the Yerevan State Medical University in Armenia reported that Schisandra chinensis, together with other adaptogen plants such as eleutherococcus and gly-cyrrhiza, protects against a particular type of fever, familial mediterranean fever. This is a condition causing fever, joint pains, muscle tenderness, rash and other signs of inflammation, which is thought to be due to a combination of genetic susceptibility and a malfunctioning immune system. The scientists studied 24 children with the condition. 14 of the children took 48 mg of the active extract of the herbal mixture every day for a period of one month, while the remaining ten children took only a placebo. At the end of the study, all of the children treated with the active mixture reported significant improvements in their symptoms, namely:

Some Adaptogenic Activities of Schisandra

• A study performed at Hong Kong University revealed that schisandrin B, obtained from the fruits of Schisandra, is a detoxifier, protecting the liver against toxic by-products of the metabolism.

• Other experiments have shown that lignans obtained from Schisandra are more powerful than vitamin E in protecting cells against free radicals.

• Schisandra extracts were able to shield cells against external chemical injury, improve the function of the cells and reduce the damage caused by lipid peroxidation, which is a dangerous and harmful biochemical reaction.

- less pain
- improved physical well-being
- reduced frequency of the fever attacks
- a less severe rash.

In addition, the results of the biochemical tests on the children treated with the active extract were all reported to have returned to normal. This, compared with the persistent symptoms and abnormal biochemical results of the children treated only with a placebo, shows that the active extract is an effective remedy against fever, inflammation and biochemical stress.

Looking at its anti-stress, or adaptogenic, activities in more detail, Japanese scientists from the Niigata College of Pharmacy found that Schisandra together with two other traditional Chinese adaptogens – Panax ginseng and Ophiopogon – can protect the brain against lack of oxygen. During a stroke or any other situation when the supply of blood to the brain is interrupted, the individual brain cells become starved of oxygen and begin to die off one by one. However, when brain cells from laboratory animals are treated with Schisandra, they become able to withstand much more punishment and can survive for longer than untreated cells. More research to see whether Schisandra improves the clinical condition of stroke patients is currently under way, but overall Schisandra is shown to be a typical and effective adaptogen, fighting stress, tiredness, memory loss, immune problems, and a poor physical condition.

Dose: The dose is 4 mg of the active extract per day. However, Schisandra is frequently found mixed with other adaptogens, as in the traditional Chinese preparation Shengmai San. There are no known contraindications or side effects.

GANODERMA

The Chinese mushroom Ling Zhi (Ganoderma lucidum) is perhaps better known as 'the mushroom of immortality'. Ancient Chinese holy men held Ling Zhi in very high regard, not only for religious and spiritual reasons, but also because of its physical properties. They believed that whoever consumes this mushroom regularly will become immortal. This may appear an outrageous claim to many people, but when scientists started looking into the medicinal properties of ganoderma they realized that there is more to this than meets the eye. While this mushroom may not make you live forever, it does have many health benefits, some of which appear truly miraculous.

One of the most important benefits of ganoderma is its cancer-fighting action. There are literally dozens of scientific experiments proving that it helps reduce the risk of cancer. In a scientific paper researchers from the Department of Medical Biochemistry at Ehime University in Japan, have shown that ganoderma blocks the growth of cancer both in the spleen and in the liver. In addition, it does not allow cancer cells to spread to other parts of the body. These researchers explained that ganoderma contains triterpenoids, which are very strong natural plant chemicals with a very important action – they destroy the blood supply to the tumour cells, thus starving these cancerous cells of oxygen and nutrients.

On the other side of the Pacific, American scientists working at the Cancer Research Laboratory of the Methodist Research Institute in Indianapolis, have shown that ganoderma, used as spores or in its dry, powdered form, blocks several chemicals which stimulate cancer to grow. Specifically, the mushroom extract blocked chemicals such as AP-1, NF-kappaB and uPA (2). These are all chemical factors which encourage cancer cells to develop and spread. So, when these chemicals are destroyed – by ganoderma, for example – the cancer cannot develop, and it withers and dies. It is not known exactly how ganoderma blocks these chemicals. Dr Sliva, who was the principal scientist in this experiment, said: 'Our data suggest that the spores and the body of Ganoderma lucidum inhibit the spread of breast and prostate cancer cells by a common mechanism, and that they would have a potential therapeutic use for the treatment of cancer.'

Another possible way that ganoderma may block cancer is by protecting the DNA. When your DNA becomes damaged by free radicals, toxins, or by ultraviolet radiation, then cancer becomes more likely. Korean scientists from the Korea Atomic Energy Research Institute have used ganoderma on cancer cells and then examined the cancerous DNA. They found that ganoderma protects the DNA against damage caused by free radicals and by radiation. Their conclusion was that the ganoderma mushroom merits further investigation as a potential preventative plant agent in cancer.

Just to expand a little further on the anti-cancer actions of ganoderma, Chinese researchers from the National Chunh-Hsing University in Taiwan have reported that it is a strong scavenger of free radicals, protecting cells and molecules alike against cancer development. This benefit is thought to be due to the high phenolic content of the mushroom. Phenolic compounds are well-known chemicals found in many plants, and are very effective at fighting free radicals.

Finally, it was also reported that ganoderma reduces the inflammatory chemical Tumour Necrosis Factor (TNF). This factor causes chronic inflammation which results in heart disease, diabetes, and dementia, and has also been implicated in cancer. Ganoderma is able to keep TNF under control and therefore the risk of cancer and also that of chronic inflammation is kept low.

Dose: The dose of the dried mushroom extract is 0.5 gm to 1 gm a day for general healthy maintenance in healthy people: 2 gm-5 gm for prevention of serious illnesses such as cancer or dementia for those who have a family history or increased risk of the disease: 5gm-10 gm a day for established illnesses, such as cancer. Up to a total of 30 gm a day has been tried without any side effects.

There are many other adaptogens, some of which can be used in combination with each other or in combination with other remedies mentioned in this book. The overall aim is to reduce the effects of stress, helping your body and mind stay healthy for longer, and thus avoiding the burden of chronic, age-related diseases.

Two Case Studies

CASE 1

A team of scientists from the Department of Urology at the College of Physicians and Surgeons in New York, has reported an intriguing case in the medical press. A man with prostate cancer proven by biopsy and microscopical examination was treated with a mixture of ganoderma and genistein. Genistein is a plant chemical commonly found in soya. The patient took this mixture once a day for six weeks, before he was due to have an operation to remove his prostate. After this six week period the doctors were amazed to see his PSA (prostatic specific antigen) blood test value fall from an initial 19.7 ng/ml to a mere 4.2 ng/ml. The PSA test is commonly used in evaluating prostate problems. Patients with prostate cancer have high PSA, while those without cancer have a low PSA. When this patient eventually had the operation to remove his prostate, there was no sign of cancer in the prostate tissue. No side effects were reported.

CASE 2

Doctors working at the Columbia-Presbyterian Medical Centre in the United States reported two other unexpected cures of patients with prostate cancer who were given ganoderma. The two men also had established cancers of their prostate proven by microscopical examination, and they were offered conventional treatment. They chose to be treated with herbal remedies instead. They took capsules of ganoderma together with other herbal remedies which work on the prostate, such as saw palmetto and scutellaria. The first patient's PSA dropped from 100 to just 24 ng/ml after a year's treatment, whereas the second patient's PSA fell from an initial 386 to a 100 ng/ml after only four months of treatment. This shows that the cancer was practically cured, or at least stopped growing.

CHAPTER 7

Calorie Restriction Mimetics

This chapter could almost be called 'How to Live Longer and be Slimmer Without Dieting'. The most reliable anti-ageing intervention which consistently increases the lifespan of animals is calorie restriction (CR). This intervention not only extends the average lifespan – the average number of years an animal is expected to live – but it also prolongs the maximum lifespan, which is the maximum number of years a particular species can possibly reach.

Different Lifespans

The maximum lifespan of mice is 3 years, while that of chimpanzees is 50 years. The human average lifespan is around 78 years, whereas the maximum human lifespan is around 110-120 years. CR also prolongs the 'health-span' which is the number of years an organism can live without any major chronic disease.

CR is also sometimes called dietary restriction and, in simple terms, is defined as under-nutrition without malnutrition. How it works is that the experimental animal is kept on a diet which consists of 30% to

70% less food than the amount consumed when there are no restrictions. The quality of the vitamins, minerals, protein, carbohydrate, fat and other ingredients in the diet is not compromised, rather it is the overall amount of calories that is reduced.

After a period of time on this diet, several age-related chemicals in the animal's blood return to normal levels and the animal looks and is healthy. Research performed at the National Institute of Aging shows that many of the beneficial effects of CR are seen not only in mice and rats but also in primates and even in humans. However, many scientists want to see more research into the effects of CR on humans before they accept its clinical benefits beyond doubt.

Scientists from the Department of Biochemistry at the University of California have reported that CR changes the activities of key enzymes, which influence the rate of protein renewal. Normally, new proteins are constantly being formed, and those damaged by free radicals, glycation, AGEs and so on are being eliminated all the time. This rate of formation and removal is balanced and fine-tuned. With age, fewer new proteins are created, while abnormal proteins are not eliminated quickly enough. The result is an excessive accumulation of damaged proteins which clog up your cells and cause further injury, contributing to the overall age-related cell malfunction. But CR can alter this state of affairs, by stimulating the creation of new proteins and speeding up the effective removal of any damaged ones. This clears up any backlog of abnormal proteins, and the cell is free to function effectively again.

CR also modulates apoptosis – orderly cell death – by modifying chaperone levels. Chaperones are molecules which take part in the formation, repair and elimination of proteins. Specifically, CR decreases the activities of chaperone molecules in the liver and increases the rate of protein elimination by up to 250%. This reduces the level of damaged proteins and improves cell function. As I will discuss later, therapeutic agents which alter the build-up of abnormal proteins, including those which reduce glycation, can be considered as having actions comparable to those of CR.

Given the fact that almost all species of animals studied so far show similar responses to CR, many anti-ageing scientists think that humans undergoing CR could also obtain benefits similar to those seen in animals. For example, their cholesterol is reduced, blood glucose levels are normalized, glucose tolerance is improved, and inflammation markers are reduced (see below). This theory received a substantial boost when results from the Biosphere 2 experiment were released. Eight scientists, who for nearly two years followed a CR regime, experienced the same physiological changes as those encountered in calorie restricted monkeys. Clearly, more human research is needed here, but the future looks promising.

CR also stimulates hormesis. This is a term referring to the long-term benefits of mild, repeated stress or stimulation. While, as explained in the previous chapter, excessive stress is bad for you, mild stresses such as increased external temperature, mild radiation exposure or nutritional stress, like CR, have been shown to improve many age-related biochemical signs. One characteristic of hormesis is that it can be activated following an event such as calorie restriction or exercise, but the results are non-proportional. In other words, mild stimulation may sometimes cause a strong effect, but at other times it may cause a weak one, depending on many other factors. This characteristic is important because it helps explain why an agent sometimes stimulates something, and why it sometimes blocks it, depending on the dose. As will be made clear later, in the case of CR there is both an inhibition of growth of cancer cells, and a stimulation of growth of healthy cells.

Biochemical and Clinical Actions of CR

Calorie restriction has the following effects. It:

reduces abnormally high blood pressure and pulse rates improves insulin activity and reduces blood glucose levels lowers body temperature, which reduces free radical damage modulates apoptosis, and improves DNA repair stimulates the production of new proteins, and the elimination of abnormal ones cuts free radicals both in numbers and in activity lowers LDL cholesterol and triglycerides and reduces body weight

increases muscle mass, and reduces fat mass

boosts DHEA production, and modulates the secretion of growth hormone

improves memory, cognition, energy, and physical activity stimulates BDNF – a nerve growth factor which benefits brain function decreases the risk of such chronic diseases as heart disease, diabetes, cancer and arthritis

There is one problem with CR however. Very few people are willing to undergo a lifetime of hunger in order to live a few extra years. Even though, according to research, CR is also effective when applied for a short period later in life, the fact remains that a few weeks or months of hunger are well beyond the capabilities of most of us in the developed world.

The good news is that 70 or so years of research into CR have not been wasted. We are now in a position to make a few educated guesses as to how exactly CR works, and try to see if we can reproduce these effects by using other, less unpalatable, interventions to achieve the same result. CR works by interfering with the activities of certain genes which produce proteins, growth factors or enzymes which, in turn, influence the rate of ageing or repair of various constituents of the body. If there was a way to influence these same genes by using a tablet or an injection, this would be a much more practical alternative than long periods of hunger and dietary discomfort.

THE GREAT IMITATORS

Calorie restriction mimetics (CRM) are drugs or chemical compounds which mimic the actions of CR. In other words, a CRM in tablet form causes the same physiological changes as CR itself. If CRM work the way they are intended to work, the big bonus in terms of human patients is that there would be no need for lengthy fasting periods. These mimetics activate biochemical pathways which are also activated by calorie restriction, and possibly by other hormetic challenges. Commonly studied mimetics are those which inhibit glycolysis (the breaking down of glucose) or those which improve the action of insulin.

One way CRM work is by affecting certain genes which ultimately cause either cell repair or cell death. For example, one gene affected by CR is the Sir2 gene in yeast. It is activated following a short period of CR and this represses the process of excessive cell death.

Apoptosis is the process whereby cells destroy themselves in response to free radicals, glycation or other toxic events, thus causing damage to the DNA. Too much apoptosis results in the loss of healthy cells which in turn causes clinical age-related symptoms.

On the other hand, too little apoptosis may result in a build-up of damaged cells which contain damaged DNA and thus contribute to cancer. Therefore a balance needs to be found between excessive and sluggish apoptosis.

One way to achieve this is through regulation and rebalancing of the excessive or sluggish activities of chemicals by using CRM. Apoptosis needs to be high in organs which regenerate easily:

- the liver
- blood
- the skin

It has to be low in organs that do not regenerate easily:

- the brain
- muscle tissues

In the first case, the risk of cancer is increased due to a quick build-up of damaged cells, so a fast rate of apoptosis is necessary in order to eliminate these damaged cells and reduce the risk of cancer. These tissues can then regenerate easily with healthy cells. In the second case, the risk of cancer is low anyway, because there is a slow turnover of cells, and any excessive apoptotic loss of cells will result in loss of function because the lost cells cannot be replaced.

The yeast Sir2 gene has an equivalent in the earthworm and, probably, in other organisms also. This has prompted scientists to look for a human equivalent and it turns out that there is a human gene similar to Sir2 which in humans is called SIRT1.

Scientists from the Department of Pathology at Harvard Medical School, have shown that low intensity stress (hormesis) such as is caused by calorie restriction, encourages SIRT1 to slow down the rate of apoptotic cell death. In this way the risk of age-related malfunction is reduced. These researchers have also shown that another gene, called PNC1 (pyrazinamide/nicotinamidase 1), stimulates an enzyme which makes the above process easier, leading to extension of the lifespan. British scientists from the Wellcome Institute at Cambridge University, have reported that the SIRT1 gene regulates factors which can modulate cell ageing.

The study of how genes are affected by CR is laborious and time-consuming. Fortunately, new technologies have managed to provide means of studying large numbers of genes at any one moment. GeneChips, which are high-density DNA microarrays, make use of technology which looks at large parts of the DNA molecule in relatively short periods of time. Workers from the Department of Biochemistry at the University of California, have reported that GeneChips can study approximately 11000 genes at any one moment. In this way it has been possible to identify several genes which may play a role in age-modification through CR. Other research companies have reported that, while a CR regime lasting two years does reverse many age-related changes, a two to four week period of CR is capable of reversing 70% of those changes. In other words, even a short CR regime lasting for up to four weeks is very effective. Genes affected in this way are those which influence inflammation, stress, apoptosis, fibrosis, and protein metabolism. Let us consider some of the CRM currently available or being tested.

METFORMIN

One of the most important CRM is the anti-diabetic drug, metformin, which modulates the activities of insulin. In order to reduce blood glucose, insulin has to be produced in sufficient amounts, but it also has to bind to insulin receptors on the cells in the body. Ageing causes increased difficulty in the smooth operation of this process, so there is a situation in which insulin cannot effectively bind to the receptors, and is unable to perform its duties properly. This is called 'increased peripheral resistance' to insulin, and it is a major factor both in diabetes and in ageing. Drugs which help mitigate this problem have existed for several years, and new ones are currently being studied.

Metformin – its brand name is Metforal – is a drug which has been in use against diabetes for over 40 years. It is considered to be a receptor sensitizer, because it enhances the sensitivity of insulin receptors on the surface of muscle and fat cells. It also increases the actual numbers of receptors. While other anti-diabetic drugs stimulate the pancreas to produce more insulin, metformin only increases sensitivity to insulin and does not influence its secretion. The upside of this is that metformin does not usually cause insulin-dependant hypoglycaemia, or hypos. When the insulin receptors are as sensitive to insulin as possible, the levels of glucose in the blood fall, fat metabolism becomes more balanced and the weight of the patient is reduced. Apart from being a receptor sensitizer, metformin also reduces glucogenesis, which is glucose production by the liver, and inhibits excessive absorption of glucose by the gut, thus contributing to the overall glucose-lowering effect.

Specifically, French researchers from the Laboratory of Endocrinology, Metabolism and Development in Paris have confirmed that metformin is able to activate genes which reduce the production of glucose by the liver, thus reducing the risk of glycation and other age-related damage. Chemical agents, such as lactate, pyruvate, alanine and galactose, can be used by the liver to create new molecules of glucose. Metformin can alter the activities of genes which make this conversion possible, reducing glucose concentration as a whole and, especially, reducing the concentration of toxic byproducts of glucose.

In addition to all this, metformin can reduce the activities of genes which increase oxidation, or free radical damage, of fatty acids. These genes contribute to the oxidation of fats which results in cell membrane disruption and eventual cell death. However, this is blocked by metformin, and it saves the cell from an early death.

At the same time, genes which produce proteins that modulate glycolysis – the destruction of glucose – are activated by metformin. It is worth remembering that CR also results in:

- the modulation of genes which affect glucose formation in the liver, so that it is high when needed, and low when it is not needed
- an influence on glycolysis or glucose elimination, which is high when energy is needed by the rest of your body, and low when it is not needed
- a containment of the glycolysis by-products which may contribute to glycation
- a lessening of AGE levels in your tissues;
- a reduction in oxidation of fatty material.

The case for metformin being a CRM is strengthened further by this.

As I mentioned above, the use of GeneChips is a quick way to test the condition of several thousand genes which may affect ageing. In an experiment, scientists tested on mice four compounds known to affect glucose metabolism. They tested the state of over 12,000 genes and found that metformin was twice as effective as the other compounds in reproducing the effects of CR. It affected a total of 63 genes, particularly those which are involved in energy production, protein formation and elimination, the growth of cells, and detoxification.

Metformin works along several different pathways, in order to control glucose activities, modulate insulin action and reduce cell death, thus increasing lifespan. However it does not always operate directly via glucose and insulin modulating pathways. It has many other 'glucose-independent' activities. With reference to hormesis metformin is able to modulate the responses to stress, so in other words it takes part in adjusting the cellular activities following mild stress.

A specific biochemical pathway is through activation of AMPK. This is an enzyme which is normally active within the cell following multiple stresses. AMPK stands for 'Adenosine Mono Phosphate-activated protein Kinase' and is, as the name suggests, activated by adenosine mono phosphate (AMP), an energy-rich molecule. Normally AMPK is switched on by stresses such as low oxygen, glucose deprivation, blocked blood supply or muscle contractions which increase the energy demands. Once activated, AMPK prevents and repairs damage to the cell, through a sudden bout of energy production and by switching off any energy-demanding processes which are not directly essential for the survival of the organism.

For example, it blocks the long-term production of proteins, fats and carbohydrates, which are not needed for the immediate survival of the cell. In other words, it behaves as if the body is in 'survival mode'. When the presence of these proteins, lipids and carbohydrates becomes essential at a later stage, once the emergency is over, then other mechanisms take over to start creating them again in the right amounts and concentrations in order to keep the cells multiplying again.

This is exactly what happens during CR when the body is in 'survival mode' and when the nutritional stress of a low calorie diet activates chemical pathways which increase the repair of cells.

Metformin and another anti-diabetic drug called rosiglitazone were shown to activate AMPK – whereas insulin blocks AMPK – and, as a result, they keep the metabolism of glucose and the state of cell repair in balance. This is important because a healthy AMPK level reflects a top heart function. It was also suggested that, by keeping AMPK active, metformin contributes to the beneficial effects of exercise which have been found in the treatment of diabetes. In addition, when metformin activates AMPK in the liver, the production of enzymes which help form new lipid molecules is reduced. Put simply, metformin through AMPK blocks the accumulation of fat.

AMPK

CR causes a mild nutritional stress with the low energy available to the cells. This stressful event activates AMPK which aims to rebalance the creation of energy, and repairs *any* cell damage (including any coincidental age-related cell damage) while switching off any processes not necessary for immediate survival. Therefore, the cell survives and the organism ultimately lives longer. Metformin, being a mimetic of CR, results in the same effect by directly activating AMPK, which confers the above benefits to the cell. The main point here is that it may not be necessary to have to undergo a period of CR to achieve cell repair, when metformin can do this itself by working on the same mechanisms as those involved in CR.

DOSAGE

Patients with kidney or liver disease, or those with heart failure should avoid taking metformin. Common and mild side effects are nausea, vomiting or abdominal bloating. The normal antidiabetic dose for metformin is 500 mg twice a day, or 850 mg daily. This can be increased as necessary to a maximum of 3000 mg a day, under medical supervision. However, the dose required for calorie restriction mimetic effects has not yet been formally calculated. In mice, a daily dose of 300 mg per kg has been shown to reduce body temperature – which is a CR mimetic effect. This cannot be extrapolated to humans, as it would mean a dose of 21000 mg for an average male! Further research is obviously needed to clarify this. Healthy people who take metformin for its general anti-ageing benefits use 500 mg twice a day.

It is important to monitor the blood biochemistry during metformin treatment. Tests commonly performed are fasting glucose and cholesterol, liver and kidney function and haemoglobin A1c, which is a glycosylated haemoglobin showing how effective the sugar levels in your body are. A low A1c means that the level of glucose, and therefore, indirectly, the level of glycation damage in your body is well controlled. Normal levels are those below the value of 5%. People who drink alcohol excessively should avoid metformin, or at least take it only under expert medical supervision.

RESVERATROL

An active plant chemical found in red wine – it comes from the skin of unripe red grapes – resveratrol has proven beneficial effects on the heart. What is more, resveratrol is a strong CRM. In yeast, it stimulates the gene Sir2, increasing the stability of DNA and extending lifespan by a good 70%. Some scientists believe that it works in the same way in humans, by activating the human gene SIRT1 which, as explained above, slows down excessive cell death in the liver, blood and skin, and reduces the risk of age-related chronic disease. Research performed at the Hormel

Institute at the University of Minnesota in the United States, shows that resveratrol has an anti-cancer activity. A derivative of resveratrol can also block cancerous cells from dividing, and thus safeguard against full-blown cancer.

A number of studies tried to discover why resveratrol sometimes speeds up apoptosis – eliminating damaged cells, keeping the risk of cancer low – and at other times blocks apoptosis – saving healthy cells from unnecessary death. The mechanisms behind this double function of resveratrol are based on hormesis as explained above, and are quite complex.

Resveratrol is normally taken in 5 mg capsules once a day for prevention, and three times a day for treatment. The dose necessary to achieve CRM effects has not been calculated but, currently, there is no reason to recommend anything other than a daily dose of 5mg to 10 mg. It is conceivable that, for a maximum CRM effect, resveratrol and metformin can be taken together or, perhaps even better, can be alternated. There is some evidence that taking medication at irregular and ever changing intervals can have a more pronounced effect on your health. However, the full efficacy of this recommendation has not yet been evaluated clinically.

An ideal way of testing the clinical benefits of the use of metformin and/or resveratrol as CRM would be to initially measure the patient's biomarkers using a computerized evaluation system (such as the Inner

Age system, see www.inner-age.com), and then to try the above treatment for a specific period of, say, six months. At the end of this period we would re-evaluate the patient's biomarkers and study the difference in the scores, particularly those related to blood glucose, insulin, cardiovascular health, liver function and brain activities, all of which might be expected to show a considerable improvement. Another way would be to use infra-red scanning to check the whole body temperature which is usually low in animals undergoing CR.

OTHER CALORIE RESTRICTION MIMETICS

There are several other, less well-known mimetics. These include chemical agents which slow down the abnormal buildup of damaged proteins in your body. Examples of these agents are aminoguanidine, carnosine and 2-deoxyglucose and they:

- prevent glycation – that abnormal binding of sugars to proteins, which, if excessive, leads to AGE formation – and therefore *prevent* AGEs
- reduce AGEs *after they are formed,* and so reduce the risk of excessive build-up of distorted proteins such as damaged collagen and elastin, and compromised enzymes, which cause several age-related clinical signs such as wrinkles, heart disease, and memory problems.

As we have observed, AGES are chemical compounds formed after glycation has already taken place. Once formed, AGEs are thought to contribute to extensive age-related damage such as the accumulation of amyloid-beta which has been implicated in Alzheimer's disease. CR reduces the concentration of AGEs and therefore helps prevent chronic disease. The same mechanism is shared by aminoguanidine and carnosine which also prevent and eliminate AGEs, and contribute towards the prevention of chronic degenerative disease.

A compound which blocks the build-up of glucose in your tissues is deoxyglucose. This has been reported to reproduce some of the effects of CR, particularly increased sensitivity of cells to insulin and reduced glucose levels as well as other biochemical changes. Research is still under way to find out more about its possible benefits for humans. What is known about 2-deoxyglucose, however, is that it can be toxic in high dosage.

CRM for the Future

Less well-researched potential CRM include the following chemicals:

hydroxycitrate which reduces appetite and caloric intake

gymnemoside which balances the metabolism of sugars

adiponectin which takes part in the metabolism of fat together with leptin which is discussed below

thiazolidinediones such as pioglitazone and rosiglitazone, which are currently used as anti-diabetic drugs

iodoacetate which protects against toxic by-products of glucose.

OTHER PROMISING MIMETICS

These are chemical factors which are still being investigated, but which have already shown promising benefits in reproducing the effects of calorie restriction. They are not available commercially, at the time of writing.

MODULATORS OF NPY

The neuropeptide Y (NPY) is a small chunk of protein which increases appetite, induces weight gain and slows down your metabolism. CR stimulates the production of NPY which encourages you to return to your normal eating habits and increase body weight. However, it is well known that the result of CR is weight loss, not weight gain. What happens is that CR selectively blocks some chemicals in the brain and stimulates others. The end result, based on hormesis is a balanced, smooth activity of CR with the known clinical benefits. Given this scientists are examining artificial ways of affecting NPY and therefore mimicking the effects of CR. An artificial chemical which re-balances the production of NPY would result in exactly the same clinical effects as those seen with CR, which works by naturally modulating NPY activity.

EXANADIN

The chemical factor exendin (exanatide) reduces the levels of glucose in your body, suppresses food intake and regulates the metabolism of sugars. It is a GLP (glucagon-like peptide) antagonist which means that it counteracts the glucose-boosting effects of the hormone glucagon. Glucagon increases blood sugar, but exanadin blocks glucagon, thus reducing blood sugar. Exanadin is a promising CRM, able to increase brain function and protect the brain against toxicity, but it is still under investigation.

THE AGENT PYY3–36

After a meal your gut releases, among other chemicals, a small piece of protein – a peptide – called PYY3-36. This then stimulates the hypothalamus, or hunger control centre, in your brain to make you stop eating. As a result, your appetite is reduced, your metabolism handles sugar better and this is considered to stimulate the same genes as those stimulated by CR. Needless to say, this chemical is still under evaluation, and it is not available commercially. When it does become available, however, it is bound to be widely used.

LEPTIN

Research performed over the past few years shows that leptin, a molecule which stimulates fat metabolism and reduces body weight, is an essential factor involved in the effects of CR. It is produced by adipocytes (fat cells) and it is involved in the response to fasting and in the hormonal changes seen during CR. Eating less causes leptin levels to fall which interferes with the production of hormones like:

- testosterone
- progesterone
- growth hormone
- thyroid hormone

Therefore, scientists believe that leptin has the same clinical effects as CR does. As a result, any chemicals that affect the production of leptin must also be classified as CRM. Together with insulin and ghrelin (a growth hormone stimulator) leptin balances the levels of appetite promoters and appetite blockers in the hypothalamus in your brain and so regulates food intake. Researchers from the Radiation Biology Branch at the Center for Cancer Research, in the National Cancer Institute at Bethesda in the United States, have shown that antioxidants influence leptin levels and so prevent obesity and the risk of cancer.

Leptin stimulates the production of AMPK and reduces the activities of enzymes which store fat. Any deficiency of or unresponsiveness to leptin, such as that seen in ageing or in obesity, causes ectopic fat accumulation, which is the storage of fat in tissues other than the white adipocytes which are those specifically designed to store fat. Ectopic fat accumulation is most obvious in the intra-abdominal tissues, which are inside your abdomen but outside your bowel. This excessive fat accumulation may cause apoptotic cell death from the pancreas and heart muscles, where ectopic fat accumulation may also take place, thus worsening diabetes and heart function. All these mechanisms show that leptin shares the same characteristics as CR and metformin.

The increased amount of research into CR has pointed us in the direction we need to take to be able to identify effective agents which reproduce the exact benefits of CR, without people having to follow long and tedious calorie-restricted diets. While research is continuing, many forward-looking doctors, who already recommend these compounds to their patients for other reasons, can now start considering the possible added bonus of the treatment.

Metformin and Leptin

These two chemicals are similar in that they both:

- aid weight loss, particularly of intra-abdominal fat, and they decrease the levels of insulin
- keep LDL (low density lipoprotein), the 'bad' type of cholesterol, at low levels
- prevent clotting, and so help reduce the risk of heart attacks and strokes
- reduce free fatty acids, triglycerides, blood pressure and appetite
- prevent glycation, cross-linking and AGEs
- improve immunity
- lower body temperature
- diminish brain damage
- stimulate BDNF, a brain-derived neurotrophic factor which is a nutrient of nerve cells
- activate AMPK

CHAPTER 8

Brain Anti-Ageing

The ageing process affects all the organs and tissues in your body, but perhaps the most important organ influenced by ageing is your brain. Many underlying biological changes that happen as we age can be seen in the brain. Oxidation, glycation, hormonal changes, inflammation, and degeneration are all present in the ageing brain, at least to a certain degree. For this reason, many doctors and scientists and other people have concentrated their efforts on finding remedies which may help prevent, slow down or even reverse some of these age-related brain changes. Although I am going to discuss some of these commonly used so-called 'brain-boosters', my aim is to offer insights into how they work during ageing, and not how they work to improve memory in healthy, young people who may want to use them during exams, for example. I will discuss in some detail one such 'brain-booster', Bacopa, which is not yet known in the wider medical community. After that I will look briefly at some other commonly used remedies or drugs.

BACOPA MONNIERI

In the wet marshlands of India grows a perennial succulent creeping herb with small green leaves.

Known in the West as 'herb-of-grace' or 'water hyssop', this plant has been mentioned in the ancient Indian medical texts from time immemorial. In Ayurvedic medicine this plant is known as the Brahmi plant – its scientific name is Bacopa monnieri. Bacopa grows in other parts of the world where there are large areas of water, and is cultivated in Florida, for example.

Ayurvedic medical practitioners use Bacopa to treat such ailments as skin infections, boils, high blood pressure, sleeping problems and water retention – fluid in the lungs, abdomen, legs or hands. The most important and well-known benefit of Bacopa, however, is in relation to brain health. Bacopa is what is known in Ayurvedic medicine as a 'rasayana'. Rasayanas are different plants which are used specifically against ageing and degeneration. They are, in other words, rejuvenating plants. In the case of Bacopa, it is used specifically against ageing of the brain, which may cause loss of memory, inability to learn new information, difficulty in thinking clearly, and general mental confusion.

Bacopa monnieri's known benefits are:

- as a brain stimulant
- as a remedy against nervous tension and stress
- for improving memory and learning
- as a general brain rejuvenator which is also possibly useful in dementia.

The two most important and well-known ingredients of Bacopa are the plant chemicals bacopaside A and bacopaside B. These are natural agents, belonging to the triterpene family of chemicals, which are widely known to be antioxidants, stimulants of the metabolism and hormone regulators. Bacopa also contains several other plant chemicals such as Bacopa saponins, which have properties similar to the bacopasides, but are not as powerful.

BRAIN HEALTH

When it comes to the brain-boosting benefits of Bacopa, there are dozens of scientific experiments proving its effectiveness. For example, in a study involving rats in the laboratory, scientists from the Central Drug Research Institute in India found that Bacopa given at a dose of 30 mg/kg, which is the equivalent of around 2000 mg in humans, significantly increases learning abilities and improves memory. In this particular study, the effects of Bacopa were examined in association with Ginkgo biloba, another well-known brain-booster. The researchers believe that both Bacopa and ginkgo work by increasing the memory-boosting chemical, acetylcholine, in the brain. Acetylcholine is a neurotransmitter which carries electrical information between the different brain cells, facilitating the consolidation of memories.

During another animal experiment, scientists from the Industrial Toxicology Research Center in Lucknow in

India, discovered exactly how Bacopa stimulates the brain and fights stress. They gave extracts of Bacopa, containing bacopasides A and B, to a group of rats, and studied the effects of this treatment on their levels of stress. The active treatment with Bacopa was tested against treatment with distilled water only. They found that the animals treated with Bacopa had a lower concentration of stress-related chemicals in their brain.

In particular, chemicals like superoxide dismutase, P450 and Hsp70, all of which go out of control when there is a stress reaction, can be restored to normal after treatment with Bacopa. When these chemicals are back within normal levels, the brain is better able to operate effectively under stress. The higher the strength of the Bacopa, the more impressive the anti-stress response. The scientists concluded that it is the bacopaside content of the extract that has these effects. This double anti-stress, memory-boosting action of Bacopa is particularly popular for people suffering from chronic brain problems, when both stress and forgetfulness need to be reduced in order to achieve a good clinical improvement.

The Benefits of Bacopa on Human Memory

A group of 76 Australians aged between 40 and 65 took part in a scientific experiment to examine the effects of Bacopa on their memory. Half of these people took Bacopa extracts at different strengths daily for three months, whereas the other half took only the dummy treatment of a placebo.

At the end of the experiment, doctors found that the people who underwent the Bacopa treatment were significantly more likely to retain new information than the placebo group were.

In addition, the Bacopa group enjoyed this benefit for six weeks after stopping the treatment. In other words, their short-term memory and recall of information did not worsen after stopping the treatment.

Further benefits of Bacopa are listed below:-

- People who have an under-active thyroid may benefit from a course of Bacopa treatment because, according to research, it stimulates the production of thyroid hormones from the thyroid gland by as much as 40%.
- Bacopa has traditionally been given to keep the stomach healthy. This effect has now been confirmed scientifically. The bacopaside A content of Bacopa is a potent anti-ulcer remedy, which helps to reduce excessive acid production in the stomach.
- Bacopa is a powerful antidepressant. When it was compared to the conventional, prescription-only antidepressant drug imipramine, Bacopa was found

to be equally as effective and without the side effects of imipramine which are a dry mouth, sleepiness, blurred vision, constipation and nausea. Bacopa is also thought to be effective against anxiety.

Dose: The active leaf extract in the purified form is available in doses of 100 mg and 300 mg to be taken daily for general brain health. In cases of marked memory problems the dose can be doubled, following advice from a health care practitioner. The raw leaf, non-purified dose is 3000 mg once or twice a day for at least four weeks.

ACETYL-L-CARNITINE

A well-known and widely used nutrient, acetyl-L-carnitine has a similar chemical structure to L – carnitine of which it is the acetylated ester. It protects the brain and nerve tissues against free radicals and other toxins. This acetylated form is better absorbed in the bowel than ordinary L-carnitine is, so it is preferred by some nutritionists.

Acetyl-L-carnitine is found in milk, and other dairy products. It is used to treat:

- depression, in association with other nutrients or drugs
- memory loss, on account of its ability to protect brain cells

- chronic brain problems, including Alzheimer's disease.

Acetyl-L-carnitine is able to shield brain cells against toxins such as excessive amounts of NMDA. As I mentioned earlier, NMDA is a brain chemical which may have an excessive activity in the brain causing excitotoxicity and leading to chronic brain degeneration.

Two other actions of acetyl-L-carnitine in the brain are its ability to protect the mitochondria where the energy production takes place, and an improvement of blood flow. This improvement in blood circulation also happens in other parts of the body. For example, acetyl-L-carnitine was found to improve intermittent claudication which is pain in the legs when walking, caused by narrow arteries.

In addition, some people have used it to protect against cataract and age-related hearing loss. This nutrient has been evaluated mainly by Italian researchers, and many British and American physicians are not convinced regarding its benefits. L-carnitine is, however, approved in the USA for use in heart disease and the lack of energy.

The side effects are mild and they include nausea, dizziness, headache and stomach upset. These are less troublesome, however, when people use a lower dose of the preparation. It may also affect sleep so it is best not to take it in the evening. Long-term effects are not yet clear. The average dose is around

500mg twice a day but this may be increased to four times a day.

ACETYL-CYSTEINE

Also called N-acetyl-cysteine, this is the acetylated form of the amino acid, cysteine. This nutrient protects your brain by stimulating the activity of glutathione, which is a potent antioxidant that protects your mitochondria from free radical damage. In addition, acetyl-cysteine may be effective against viruses and it is used both for prevention and treatment of some viral infections, including brain infections. It protects the liver from damage and helps loosen up thick mucus. Conventional doctors use acetyl-cysteine to counteract the consequences of paracetamol overdose. It is also found in some cough mixtures. Patients who are on nitrates, such as GTN spray or isosorbide for heart problems, may experience an improved effect from their medication, because acetyl-cysteine helps nitrates stay active in the body.

Dose: The normal dose is 500 mg, once or twice a day for cysteine, and around 1000 mg-1500mg a day for acetyl-cysteine. Some doctors recommend that people also take vitamin C supplements when taking acetyl-cysteine to prevent it from being destroyed in the body prematurely.

ALPHA LIPOIC ACID

This is another antioxidant which also boosts the levels of glutathione in your body. It is an essential factor in reactions involving the production of energy in your cells. It is both water and fat soluble, which means that it can easily reach most parts of the body. Alpha lipoic acid works together with vitamins C and E, strengthening their actions.

It is used in treating diabetic complications and to generate energy in the mitochondria. It helps in the elimination of toxic metals and protects against excessive glycation. Overall, it is believed to be effective at improving memory, brain function and learning, but most of the studies have been performed on animals in the laboratory, and not on human patients.

Dose: The recommended dose is from 20 mg– 250mg daily. Many commercial preparations offer alpha lipoic acid together with acetyl-L-carnitine because some laboratory experiments have shown that the two work better if given together in one dose, rather than separately.

CENTROPHENOXINE

Many European doctors prescribe centrophenoxine to treat a range of brain problems such as failing memory and mental tiredness. Centrophenoxine is used to boost brain energy, increasing the brain’s use of oxygen and glucose. It is also used in the treatment of age-related damage to the brain, and for stroke, injury or drug damage. Experiments show it to increase memory and learning capabilities both in laboratory animals and in humans.

From an experiment performed at the School of Life Sciences at Nehru University in India, scientists concluded that centrophenoxine activates the brain enzyme called acetyl-cholinesterase, which takes part in regulating memory. The scientists found that the activity of this enzyme falls with age, and this is particularly noticeable in the memory centres of the brain, the hippocampus. Centrophenoxine supplements were able to stop this decline and restore acetylcholinesterase levels to youthful ones.

Treatment with centrophenoxine produces other benefits:

- It reduces the levels of lipofuscin which is a waste material found in the brains and muscles of aged organisms.
- It stimulates the production of RNA which is essential for top brain performance.
- It was found to increase lifespan in laboratory animals.
- It may strengthen the effects of other brain-boosters such as hydergine or piracetam.

Professor Imre Zs-Nagy of the University of Debrecen in Hungary, a well-respected anti-ageing expert, believes that free radicals make the cells very vulnerable to damage, resulting in brain and memory problems. Centrophenoxine is able to protect against this type of damage by boosting the activity of other antioxidants inside the cell. He has developed a newer and stronger variant of centrophenoxine, called BCE-001 which is still under scrutiny by scientists.

Dose: The dose of centrophenoxine is 250mg twice a day, with regular breaks. It should not be taken by those who have epilepsy or those with severe high blood pressure. It may also cause nausea, dizziness and muscle stiffness.

DEPRENYL

Also known as selegiline, deprenyl stops the destruction of dopamine, a chemical which is low in sufferers from Parkinson's disease. In this way, deprenyl increases the concentration of dopamine in the brain which is important because healthy amounts of dopamine – neither too high, nor too low – are essential in normal brain function, both with regards to memory and to co-ordination of movements. Doctors who support the use of deprenyl say that it banishes depression and mental stress, increases libido and improves the quality of life in Alzheimer's or Parkinson's disease patients. Conventional doctors use it as a standard treatment for Parkinson's disease.

Some people have reported that it also improves the sense of touch.

Deprenyl has extended the lifespan of laboratory animals in certain experiments, which is why some people use it as a general anti-ager. There are many research reports supporting the use of deprenyl in different brain conditions. Overall, the research confirms that deprenyl is a brain protector improving the transmission of information from one part of the brain to another. Not only does it activate dopamine, but it also boosts the activity of another brain chemical, noradrenaline. These two work in unison, in a balanced manner, to achieve smooth, co-ordinated movements and better memory in patients. Experiments show that deprenyl prevents apoptosis, which if left uncontrolled leads to dementia and other chronic brain diseases.

Dose: The liquid form is thought to be better absorbed than the tablets. Liquid deprenyl is taken sublingually (under the tongue). The dose depends on the condition which is being treated: Parkinson's and Alzheimer's sufferers have been known to use 10mg-20 mg daily. Used against ageing, the dose is 2.5mg-5mg twice a week, under medical supervision. Older patients may need to use higher doses according to their age. It should not be taken by people who are already taking antidepressants or anaesthetics. Side effects are nausea, dizziness, confusion, stomach pains and vivid dreams. Brand names for deprenyl are Eldepryl and Jumex.

HYDERGINE

Like centrophenoxine, hydergine is a chemical which reduces lipofuscin deposits in the brain and improves brain metabolism. It is an antioxidant and 'smart drug' derived originally from rye, and is used quite extensively by some European and Asian doctors. There are several chemical members related to hydergine, all of which belong to the ergot family, called ergoloid mesylates.

Hydergine protects the brain against toxic damage and improves the connections between brain cells (dendrites). It also stimulates the action of brain neurotransmitters, which facilitate the flow of information within your brain. Hydergine may reduce a destructive molecule, called senescent cell antigen, which is found in old cells.

A group of scientists working at the National Institute of Mental Health in Maryland in the United States examined all the available data – both positive and negative – about hydergine. They knew that hydergine is used for treating patients with dementia or age-related memory problems, yet the scientific proof of its efficacy was uncertain. They found a total of 19 experiments which were rigorous enough to be analyzed. Their conclusions were that hydergine has an overall positive effect on dementia, with no significant side effects. However, most of the research was relatively old, having been performed in the early

80s when the standards for evaluating dementia were not as tight as they are currently. Nevertheless, more modern experiments show hydergine to be able to improve learning and memory in experimental animals.

Dose:-The dose varies from 3 mg to10 mg daily. It is available in tablet and liquid form. Side effects include nausea and stomach upset which again should respond to a lowering of the dose.

RESVERATROL

Resveratrol is a polyphenol found mainly in the skin of red grapes. Significant amounts are also found in peanuts. Apart from its actions as a calorie restriction mimetic, outlined in the previous chapter, resveratrol also helps lower the likelihood of cancer by reducing the concentration of carcinogens (chemicals which cause cancer), blocking the growth of cancer cells and stimulating the immune system. It can also help reduce the risk of heart disease and is an antioxidant and blocks abnormal blood clotting, as well as reducing the damage caused by LDL (the 'bad' cholesterol). Its benefits on the brain are due to its ability to improve blood supply to the brain cells, and protect them against free radicals.

Resveratrol may interact with other blood-thinning medication such as aspirin, warfarin and ginkgo biloba, and should not be used by people with blood clotting abnormalities. It is available in tablet form in doses between 5mg and 30 mg.

Research shows that a diet supplemented with resveratrol, as well as with other antioxidants such as vitamins C and E, N-acetylcysteine, deprenyl, alpha lipoic acid and co-enzyme Q10 protects the mitochondria inside your cells and improves the process of energy production which ensures a longer lifespan. This confirms that it may be better to take several different supplements which work in unison with each other for a more powerful result.

VINPOCETINE

The periwinkle plant (Vinca minor) has been used by traditional medical healers for many centuries to deal with mental problems. It invigorates the brain function and metabolism, and works by blocking sodium movements across the cell membrane as it is a sodium channel blocker. This helps in certain steps of the chemical signalling between nerve cells. Vinpocetine improves the use of oxygen by the brain, improving the availability of energy.

Vinpocetine increases the levels of ATP which is the molecule needed for the production of energy. It protects the brain against lack of oxygen in cases of reduced blood flow in the brain arteries, and it also improves blood supply. It is used with some benefit in certain cases of stroke and brain injury. It is also used to prevent stroke or brain ageing, as well as dizziness, vertigo, tinnitus, and depression. There have been some experiments the results of which endorse these uses but many conventional doctors remain sceptical about it.

Dose: The dose is 5 mg three times a day. Side effects are rare but include fast heart beat and low blood pressure which improves once the dose is adjusted. There are no known toxic reactions or problems with interactions with other drugs.

Several other 'brain-boosters' or nootropics are available commercially. It is important to have a medical assessment before you decide to take any of these, in order to establish with your practitioner exactly what your aims are and how the particular medication may be expected to help you. Also, do remember that although many people have reported positive benefits after taking these remedies, many others have not noticed any difference in their brain abilities at all.

CHAPTER 9

Living Longer

Taking pills and supplements to try to reduce the signs of ageing is only the beginning. If you want to increase your chances of living a healthy, active life for as long as possible you should also explore other ways of achieving this aim, apart from taking pills.

Regular exercise is one of the most efficient ways of overcoming a number of age-related problems. Remember, however, that too much exercise, lasting over 45 minutes at a time, may actually fuel the production of free radicals and so it should be avoided. The best exercises to keep your body really fit are:

- swimming
- brisk walking
- dancing
- light gym exercises
- aerobics
- gentle weight lifting
- Oriental exercises such as yoga, tai chi and chi kung.

Suitable nutrition should also be high on your agenda. I have discussed anti-ageing nutrition extensively in some of my other books (*Stay Young Longer – Naturally,* and *The Age Defying Cookbook).* Suffice it to say that, due to questions raised about the nutrient content of our modern diet, it is increasingly becoming recognized amongst nutritionists that we need to supplement our diet with extra nutritional supplements in tablet form.

I have mentioned many times that all anti-ageing treatments are a matter of balance. The same is true of our diet. You should try and strike a balance between gorging yourself on foods that you do not like but which are good for you, and having enough freedom to enjoy your life without too many unpleasant restrictions on the food you consume.

In addition to good nutrition and exercise, mental attitudes and positive thinking are also essential in fighting ageing. There is no point in taking a few pills and doing some exercise, when your brain remains neglected, and your thoughts become stale. You need to see growing older as a bonus rather than as a burden. Your aim should be to face ageing straight on, but to maintain as many characteristics of youth as possible, and this includes a good, effective brain and a positive mental outlook. I have discussed all of these aspects in detail in previous books.

It is important to realize that nutrition, mental and physical exercises, and anti-ageing medication need to be used together, so we make a continuing effort through our lifestyle to defeat problems related to ageing for as long as possible. You should constantly question the things you do for your health, see if they can be improved and keep an eye on new developments which may help you.

However, do not be fooled by false or sensational advertising or claims. Ask to see the proof behind each product and, if there is no proof that it works, ask yourself whether you want to try it and see, or move on to something else more promising.

Here are two examples to illustrate how effective anti-ageing medication can be in certain aspects of everyday life.

CASE NUMBER 1

Two married couples in their seventies decided to experiment with carnosine. Both couples were doing approximately the same amount of exercise and ate the same kind of diet and followed a similar lifestyle. One member of each couple took 50 mg of carnosine a day for four months whereas their partner did not.

Their party trick was to ask their friends and relatives to guess who was on carnosine and who was not. The funny thing was that most of the time their friends and relatives guessed correctly. This shows you that, no matter what research says, some supplements can indeed have a noticeable impact on whether an individual actually looks healthier or not. Whether the supplement in question truly changes things inside you is a different matter. It may or it may not. How you look, how you feel and what other people think about your appearance is, however, very relevant in life.

CASE NUMBER 2

One of my patients, a woman aged 45 was using over 80 different tablets and capsules a day, as well as doing a lot of exercise trying to keep fit. She considered herself to be very healthy and 'in the know' regarding health matters. However, after undergoing some blood tests and anti-ageing computerized assessments she discovered that her scores were surprisingly bad.

The amount of medication she was taking was not really relevant to ageing, and her exercise regime was excessive. She did not pay any attention to the health of her brain but wanted to remain young at all costs, hating the idea of getting chronologically older.

Following a selective reduction of her medication and a decrease in exercise time, she also underwent a series of counselling sessions to learn how to cope with her increasing age, and to see her own ageing as a natural and healthy part of life. She was of course started on carnosine 100 mg–150 mg a day, as well as DHEA, Q10 and SAMe. After six months of this treatment, her computerized scores improved considerably, and all her detailed blood and urine tests were completely normal.

This highlights one of the most important and frequently neglected aspects of anti-ageing medicine, that it is necessary to use a holistic approach to deal with any problems and not try to deal with problems individually.

FIGHTING AGEING FROM WITHIN

A new way which can be taken to delay certain signs of ageing is based on a mathematical theory called the theory of dynamical systems, which is more commonly known as chaos theory. This is how it works. Your body is very complex and contains a vast amount of biological reserves. Just consider that you are probably using only 10% of your brain's potential at any given time, keeping the other 90% in reserve. The same is true for many other organs and processes in your body. This degree of complexity gradually declines with age, resulting in chronic disability, illnesses and your body's general inability to function properly until life becomes impossible and death occurs.

According to chaos theory, because life is based on complexity, and because loss of this complexity equals ageing and death, then an increase in complexity must equal health. So, if there was a way to increase this complexity, it would be possible to prevent and reverse some of the age-related decline, increasing your reserves which can then be called on when necessary.

In a research paper entitled 'Practical Applications of Chaos Theory to the Modulation of Human Ageing: nature prefers chaos to regularity' (*Biogerontology* 2003:4(2):75-90), I applied mathematical concepts to devise several practical exercises which can be used to increase the complexity in your body.

The most important step in this context is to increase the amount of innovation and the input of new information in your life. You need to avoid regular and boring activities which fail to keep your body and mind active and stimulated. Routine, sameness and boredom in your life do not contribute to health.

Any type of stimulation – physical, mental, social, sensual and spiritual – should be used, in order to keep your body and mind agile and energetic, and I offer some suggestions for you to consider below.

PHYSICAL STIMULATION

Day 1. Do 30 minutes tai chi in the morning and 20 minutes ballroom dancing in the evening.

Day 2. Go for a 20 minute brisk walk, and then do 15 minutes yoga.

Day 3. Play football or other ball games for 30 minutes in the afternoon.

Day 4. No exercise, just follow your everyday routine.

Day 5. Try a new sport, such as horse riding, fencing or rowing.

Day 6. Go to the gym for 20-25 minutes of weight lifting.

Day 7. Practise some aerobics for 30 minutes, followed by some yoga.

Day 8. No exercise, but keep generally active.

MENTAL STIMULATION

- Choose a controversial subject and then argue the case against the opinion you hold about it.
- Try listening to unusual music, such as traditional oriental songs.
- Tune into a foreign-language radio station and try to guess the general meaning of the programme you are listening to.
- For about 5-10 minutes try and read a magazine holding it upside down. To make the exercise more difficult, hold it upside down in front of a mirror and then try reading from the mirror image.

- Lie on the floor for 10 minutes and examine your surroundings from this unusual view point.
- For 5-10 minutes a day use your non-dominant hand to write something.
- Read a magazine or a newspaper that you do not usually read.

SOCIAL AND SPIRITUAL STIMULATION

- Do not accept easy answers or explanations. Always look for the real reason behind any event or situation that you take part in.
- Find a way of strengthening your social bonds, your friendships and your family ties.
- Take an active part in your society, by volunteering to help with local projects or doing charity work.
- Explore other religions.
- Explore aspects of your own religion which you have not considered in the past.

NUTRITIONAL STIMULATION

Apart from a calorie restricted regime which is not currently recommended in everyday situations, below is another example of nutritional stimulation.

If you are taking vitamins, or herbal or nutritional supplements it could be better to try and take them at irregular intervals instead of taking the same dose every day at a regular time. For instance, on one day you could take your vitamin E in the morning, your vitamin C before lunch, your co-enzyme Q10 tablets in the afternoon and your glucosamine in the evening. The next day you could take only two of the above together and one at night, missing one out. The day after that do not take anything. The day after take one of the above at lunchtime and the three others in the afternoon. And so on. I would emphasize that you should, however, only do this under expert supervision.

With regards to nutrition, it is well known that consuming a variety of foodstuffs and eating small and frequent meals is beneficial to health. Try to alternate your meals and include unusual foods which are not normally part of your diet such as exotic fruit, game, or nuts.

By following a carefully planned, but irregular and apparently haphazard lifestyle, you increase the amount of meaningful stimulation to your body and mind, therefore lending a hand in maintaining the complex biological reserves of your body. This may help you ward off ageing and disability. Although, to an untrained observer, what you are doing may appear chaotic, it should in fact be planned very carefully with logic behind each step.

Many of the treatments discussed in this book only affect certain aspects of ageing, and questions still remain as to whether other aspects of the ageing process can be stopped completely or even reversed. However, a combination of suitable medication with a healthy lifestyle can go a long way in helping you through the ageing process.

What matters is you. If you feel satisfied with a particular nutrient or drug, if you enjoy your lifestyle and if you are content with your plan of action, then so be it. We only have a comparatively short time on this earth and we should make the most of it. But also remember that you can influence that time, to a certain degree. Choose wisely and you will increase it both in quality and in quantity. Choose poorly, and you will make it even shorter. It's up to you.

Glossary

Adaptogens – plant remedies which help the body to adapt to chronic stress

Alzheimer's dementia– an age-related form of brain damage resulting in severe forgetfulness, inability to look after oneself, cognition problems and disorientation

Antioxidants – substances which reduce or fight free radicals

Apoptosis – the 'falling off of cells. It is a natural type of orderly and programmed cell death which eliminates damaged cells while leaving healthy cells behind untouched. It is the opposite of 'necrosis' which is a disorderly and widespread cell death.

Atherosclerosis – the thickening of the inside part of the arteries which is in contact with the blood. Fatty deposits, small blood clots and other by-products of inflammation may block the flow of blood.

Calorie restriction mimetics – drugs or supplements which have similar biological effects to the restriction of calories

Cross-over study – half of the participants in the study are given the real treatment to be tested, and the other half are given a placebo. After a certain time, the two groups change over and those who were taking the placebo are given the active treatment, while those who were taking the active treatment receive the placebo. The result of this study gives a better idea of the effectiveness of the tested treatment.

DNA– Deoxyribonucleic acid. This is a long string of chemicals, like a complicated step-ladder, containing all the genetic information necessary for the production of another organism similar to the original.

Double-blind study – a study in which neither the investigator nor the patient knows whether the patient is receiving active treatment or just a placebo. This ensures that the results are as independent as possible. A third party checks the results.

Hormone – a chemical messenger compound, produced and released into the bloodstream by endocrine organs (glands). Examples of hormones are: insulin, DHEA, GH, oestrogen, progesterone, testosterone, pregnenolone, melatonin.

Molecule – a chemical structure with individual chemical properties. Examples of molecules are proteins, DNA, enzymes, free radicals, sugars, aldehydes etc.

Pituitary gland – a small gland secreting several hormones, located on the midline towards the base of the brain.

Placebo – dummy treatment. A placebo-controlled study is one which compares the effects of some proper treatment against the effects of placebo.

Platelets – blood constituents which take part in the clotting of the blood. A high activity of platelets causes increased clotting, whereas a low activity may result in haemorrhage.

Pro-oxidants – substances which enhance oxidation.

Further Reading

Coenzyme Q10 Phenomenon, Dr S Sinatra, Keats Publishing, Connecticut, 1998

DHEA Breakthrough, S A Cherniske, Ballantine Books, New York, 1997

Grow Young with HGH, R Klatz, HarperCollins, New York, 1997 (For more information regarding secretagogue products see www.antiaginginfo.net/compare.htm)

Methyl Magic, Craig Cooney, Andrews McMeel Publishing, Kansas City, 1999

Stay Young, Longer – Naturally, Dr Marios Kyriazis, Vega, London, 2001

Useful Addresses

SUPPLIERS OF DRUGS AND SUPPLEMENTS

In the USA and other parts of the world:– International Anti-aging Systems (including the Far East), Life Extension Foundation, Vitamin Research Products (for addresses, see below).

In the UK:– The Nutricentre, 7 Park Crescent, London W1N 3HE, tel.: 020 7436 5122, www.nutricentre.co.uk

In Australia:– www.betaalistine.com.au

Also from: www.smart-drugs.com www.integratedhealth.com www.artemisherbs.co.uk

Vespro Ltd:– The suppliers of the Free Radical Kit www.vespro-europe.co.ukwww.vesproeurope.comwww.vespro.com

ORGANISATIONS

The British Longevity Society:–This is a UK-based organisation which aims to inform the general public about the latest news in the field of anti-ageing medicine. It is where I can be contacted.

P.O. Box 71, Hemel Hempstead, HP3 9DN United Kingdom www.antiage.org.uk email: kyriazis@antiageing.freeserve.co.uk

International Anti-Aging Systems (IAS):– IAS are a global organisation, the sponsors and organisers of the Monte Carlo Anti-Aging Conference. They publish regular bulletins, catalogues and directories, but they are unable to deliver to UK addresses.

Les Autelets, Sark GY9 0SF, Channel Islands, UK tel.: 01144 8701514144 www.antiaging-systems.com

The Life Extension Foundation:– Members receive a monthly magazine with the latest information on all aspects of ageing. The Foundation also offers many other resources and products. P.O. Box 229120, Hollywood, Florida 33022-9120, USA www.lef.org

VRP (Vitamin Research Products):– They are a US-based company offering a variety of products, including carnosine. 3579 Hwy 50 East, Carson City, Nevada 89701 USA tel.: 800 877 2447

www.vrp.com

email: mail@vrp.com

World Wide Health Corporation:– They can supply products and anti-ageing information.

WWH, Alderney GY1 5SS, UK

www.wwh-corp.com

American Academy of Anti-aging Medicine:– Some academics do not recognize this as an official organisation, but it does organize an annual conference on anti-ageing. It issues the *International Journal of Anti-Aging Medicine,* and other related publications. It runs an accreditation program for qualifications in anti-aging medicine, and has a record of practitioners from around the world.

1341 W Fullerton, Suite 111, Chicago IL 60614, USA
tel.: 773 528 43330

www.worldhealth.net

Printed in Dunstable, United Kingdom

91226153R00127